Foreword

Surely as human beings we all experience defining moments in our lives when something changes forever how we see ourselves and our world. For me one such moment occurred while being taught by the paediatrician Ronnie McKeith, a very unusual man in many respects who devoted his professional life to improving the assessment and care of children with cerebral palsy. During our three months of paediatrics a small group of us would gather in his study once a week for a seminar. The content and direction of the teaching was utterly unpredictable and no doubt contrary to more recent educational theory. There were certainly no learning objectives defined at the outset. On this occasion he passed around a photograph of an infant with some vague invitation to comment on what we saw. We made various suggestions – was the child anaemic, hypocalcaemic, did the ears indicate some syndrome? Eventually he had to tell us: the baby was dead. It was lying with its head at an unnatural angle, on a mortuary table with a white tiled wall behind, and dressed in a shroud. His point was that already, as medical students, we had found a means of pushing out of our considerations and out of our conscious minds, the inevitable final outcome of all our medical care – death.

The single life event that will be experienced by all living creatures is that someday we will die. There are no exceptions. This report draws our attention to the plain fact that for most of us our death will be in an acute hospital under circumstances which were not set up to ensure peace, privacy, dignity, and the gathering of a family in the way they would choose – which would be the priorities in allowing natural death. Instead the modern hospital has processes in place to ward off death. Time is of the essence. A team gathers around the bed. Orders are given and received. Nurses, doctors and technicians are all geared up to respond rapidly with heart massage and electric shocks. Cannulae are inserted into veins and arteries. A tube is put in to assist breathing - plus any number of other intrusions and connections to medical kit.

It should be remembered that the report is based around a collection of case histories of people who died, comprising technical documentation and medical narratives. Some were not expected to die and for them the emphasis is on identifying any elements in their care which might have been better handled. For others death was the expected outcome, either from the outset or after initial assessment.

What comes out vividly in the report is the challenge we face as medical teams in making the transition between saving life and allowing natural death, two entirely appropriate but conflicting objectives. To do this at the right time and to ensure that the change is made with the informed consent of those most concerned - the dying person and those they would prefer to have near. The report does not suggest that there are easy answers and I will do no better in my foreword but there are some social and cultural expectations placed on modern medical practice which are highlighted.

The authors of the report draw a comparison between the usual death a century ago and what happens now. Back then cardiac and respiratory arrest were irreversible, pneumonia was referred to as the old man's friend, and severe bleeding and kidney failure were commonly fatal, whereas we now expect all of these to be recoverable. When Ronnie McKeith taught us in the 1960s the few intensive care beds at Guy's were in the hands of the cardiac surgeons and coronary surgery and angioplasty were not yet on the scene. Modern medicine has been hugely successful in blocking one after another of the too early routes of exit but, perhaps partly as a consequence of being able to postpone the inevitable so successfully in so many instances, a timely death remains difficult to discuss and therefore perhaps less well managed than it might be.

Professor T Treasure
NCEPOD Chairman

Principal findings

In 25% (407/1635) of cases there was, in the view of the advisors, a clinically important delay in the first review by a consultant.

Poor communication between and within clinical teams was identified by the advisors as an important issue in 13.5% (267/1983) of cases.

There was a lack of communication both between different grades of doctors within clinical teams, and between different clinical teams and other health care professionals.

There were instances of poor decision making and lack of senior input, particularly in the evenings and night time.

95.8% of these sick patients were anaesthetised by an anaesthetist of the appropriate grade for their condition.

Access to CT scanning and MRI scanning is a substantial problem with many sites having no or limited (<24hours) on site provision.

Only 150/297 hospitals have on site angiography (non-cardiac) and of these only 76 have 24 hour access.

District hospitals may have particular problems delivering a high standard of care when dealing with very sick children and it is recognised that a well co-ordinated team approach is required.

In 16.9% (219/1293) of patients who were not expected to survive on admission there was no evidence of any discussion between the health care team and either the patient or relatives on treatment limitation.

In 21.8% of cases DNAR orders were signed by very junior trainee doctors.

There were examples of where health care professionals were judged not to have the skills required to care for patients nearing the end of their lives. This was particularly so in relation to a lack of the abilities to identify patients approaching the end of life, inadequate implementation of end of life care and the poor communication with patients, relatives and other health care professions.

Introduction

Following the admission of patients in an emergency or urgent setting there is often no formal assessment of comorbidities. Many, otherwise remediable, medical conditions go uncorrected, problems are overlooked, surgical complication rates are high and deaths occur despite the best anaesthetic, surgical and medical expertise available[1].

Much can be done to pre-empt such problems but this requires good planning and service and a team that functions in a co-ordinated manner. Continuity of care and an understanding of the case throughout the patient's hospital stay must be assured. Change in the hospital team structure over recent years has seen individual clinicians become transient acquaintances during a patient's illness rather than having responsibility for continuity of care. Staffing arrangements and shift working have also been shown to be disruptive[1] and with the implementation of the European Working Time Directive, this disruption is likely to continue and to impact on the training of tomorrow's doctors.

Better team working involves consultants and all medical staff working together with nurses, managers and professions allied to medicine and sometimes patients themselves. It is possible that emergency situations may not allow this way of working but, with time and effective communication, specialist groups should be able to anticipate and plan for most common scenarios of presentation and the associated complications. This can be seen clearly in the paediatric section of this report and in the end of life care section. More patients are dying in hospital and it should be ensured that patients achieve the best quality of life until they die. Effective team working and communication with patients, relatives and carers are fundamental to getting this right.

The study presented in this report revisits some of the themes highlighted in the 2002[1], 2003[2] and 2007[3] NCEPOD reports, to evaluate current practice and see what changes have been made.

1 - Method

Study aim

To explore remediable factors in the process of care for patients who died in an hospital.

Objectives

The expert group identified objectives that would address the overall aim of the study and these will be addressed throughout the following chapters:
- assessing process of referral from admission until seen by first consultant;
- handover and multidisciplinary team working;
- levels of supervision;
- appropriateness of surgery and anaesthesia;
- general clinical issues including prophylaxis for venous thromboembolism and access to investigations including radiology services;
- paediatric practice;
- palliative care in an acute setting.

Hospital participation

National Health Service hospitals in England, Wales and Northern Ireland were expected to participate, as well as hospitals in the independent sector and public hospitals in the Isle of Man, Guernsey and Jersey.

Within each hospital, a named contact, referred to as the NCEPOD Local Reporter, acted as a link between NCEPOD and the hospital staff, facilitating case identification, dissemination of questionnaires and data collation.

Study population

All patients older than 28 days who died in hospital between 1st October 2006 and 31st March 2007 within 96 hours of admission were included.

Exclusion criteria

Neonates under 28 days old.

Case ascertainment

The NCEPOD Local Reporter identified all patients who died within their hospital(s) during the study period, regardless of disease type or disorder. The information requested for each case included the primary and secondary diagnosis codes and details of the clinician responsible for the patient at the time of death.

Questionnaires and case notes

There were three questionnaires used to collect data for this study, a clinical questionnaire per patient which covered all aspects of patient care during their admission. If the patient had received an anaesthetic then an anaesthetic questionnaire was sent to the anaesthetist involved. For each site, completion of an organisational questionnaire was requested. This questionnaire concerned data on the staff, facilities and protocols available to care for patients in hospital.

The organisational questionnaire was sent to the NCEPOD Local Reporter for completion in collaboration with relevant specialty input. Clinical questionnaires were either sent to the NCEPOD Local Reporter for dissemination or directly to the consultant clinician involved. However, whichever method was used, it was requested that the completed questionnaires were returned directly to NCEPOD to maintain confidentiality.

For each case to be peer reviewed photocopies of the following case note extracts were requested:
- inpatient annotations;
- nursing notes;
- haematology and biochemistry results;
- drug charts;
- fluid balance charts (including urine output)
- observation charts;
- weight chart;
- urinalysis;
- x-ray/CT/ultrasound results;
- any operating notes;
- do not attempt resuscitation statement;
- autopsy report.

Advisor group

A multidisciplinary group of advisors was recruited to review the case notes and associated questionnaires. The group of advisors comprised clinicians from all specialties, both medical and surgical.

All questionnaires and case notes were anonymised by the non-clinical staff at NCEPOD. All patient, clinician and hospital identifiers were removed. Neither clinical co-ordinators at NCEPOD, nor the advisors had access to any information that could be used to identify individual patients, staff or hospitals.

After being anonymised each case was reviewed by one advisor within a multidisciplinary group. At regular intervals throughout the meeting, the chair allowed a period of discussion for each advisor to summarise their cases and ask for opinions from other specialties or raise aspects of a case for discussion.

The grading system below was used by the advisors to grade the overall care each patient received.

> **Good practice:** A standard that you would accept from yourself, your trainees and your institution.
> **Room for improvement:** Aspects of *clinical* care that could have been better.
> **Room for improvement:** Aspects of *organisational* care that could have been better.
> **Room for improvement:** Aspects of both *clinical* and *organisational* care that could have been better.
> **Less than satisfactory:** Several aspects of clinical and/or organisational care that were well below that you would accept from yourself, your trainees and your institution.
> **Insufficient information submitted to NCEPOD to assess the quality of care.**

Quality and confidentiality

Each case was given a unique NCEPOD number so that cases could not easily be linked to a hospital.

The data from all questionnaires received were electronically scanned into a preset database. Prior to any analysis taking place, the data were cleaned to ensure that there were no duplicate records and that erroneous data had not been entered during scanning. Any fields that contained spurious data that could not be validated were removed.

Data analysis

Following cleaning of the quantitative data, descriptive data summaries were produced.

The qualitative data collected from the advisors' opinions and free text answers in the clinical questionnaires were coded, where applicable, according to content to allow quantitative analysis. The data were reviewed by NCEPOD clinical co-ordinators to identify the nature and frequency of recurring themes.

Case studies have been used throughout this report to illustrate particular themes.

All data were analysed using Microsoft Access and Excel by the non-clinical staff at NCEPOD.

The findings of the report were reviewed by the expert group, advisors and the NCEPOD steering group prior to publication.

2 - Data returns

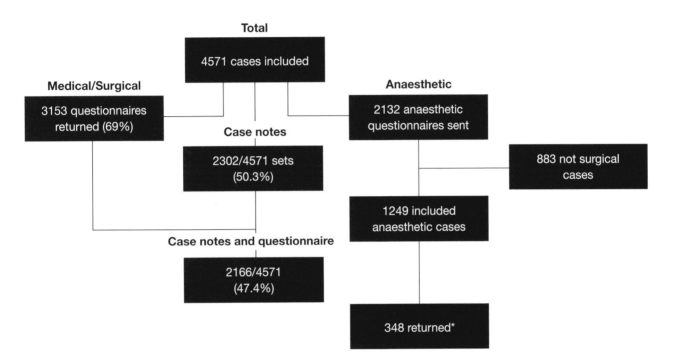

Total

4571 cases included

Medical/Surgical

3153 questionnaires returned (69%)

Anaesthetic

2132 anaesthetic questionnaires sent

883 not surgical cases

Case notes

2302/4571 sets (50.3%)

1249 included anaesthetic cases

Case notes and questionnaire

2166/4571 (47.4%)

348 returned*

Figure 2.1 Data returns

*An anaesthetic questionnaire was sent for all cases where a patient had undergone a medical or surgical procedure. This was determined from the OPCS codes provided on the initial case data sent to NCEPOD. If no OPCS code was present an anaesthetic questionnaire was also sent for all cases admitted under a surgical specialty, anaesthetic specialty or emergency medicine. However, this meant that determining the true denominator for the anaesthetic questionnaire has not been possible and so we have not presented a percentage return rate.

Study sample denominator data by chapter

Within this study the denominator will change for each chapter and occasionally within each chapter. This is because data has been taken from different sources depending on the analysis required. For example in some cases the data presented will be a total from a question taken from the clinical questionnaire only, whereas some analysis may have required the total for one question from the clinical questionnaire to be crossed with the advisors' view taken from the case notes. As there were more clinical questionnaires than case notes the complete data included will be less. A table giving a summary of the denominators used will be provided at the start of each section.

3 - Study population and overall quality of care

		Denominator
Clinical questionnaire	Total population	3153
Assessment form	Total population	2302

Age and gender

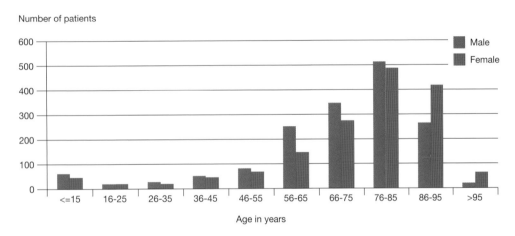

Figure 3.1 Age distribution of patients in this study by gender

Most of the population examined in this study was elderly, with a majority of patients admitted aged 66 or over; 49% of the patients admitted were male and 51% female with a median age of 77 (range 0 – 105) (Figure 3.1).

Just over half of patients were admitted under a physician and just under half under the care of a surgeon (Table 3.1). (Paediatrics has been counted as a medical specialty; obstetrics and gynaecology as a surgical specialty).

Specialty of admitting clinician

Table 3.1 Specialty of admitting clinician

Specialty	n	%
Medical	1521	52.7
Surgical	1364	47.3
Subtotal	**2885**	
Not answered	268	
Grand Total	**3153**	

Mode of admission

Table 3.2 Pathway for admission

Pathway	n	%
Admission via emergency department	1772	56.6
Referral from general medical or dental practitioner	597	19.0
Admission following a previous outpatient consultation	140	4.5
Planned re-admission/routine follow up procedure	28	<1
Unplanned re-admission following day case or outpatient procedure	10	<1
Unplanned admission following day case or outpatient procedure	20	<1
Transfer as an inpatient from another hospital	221	7.1
Walk in clinic	4	<1
Tertiary (same specialty)	19	<1
Tertiary (other specialty)	7	<1
Self referral by patient	101	3.2
Transferred from a nursing or residential home	56	1.8
Other	137	4.4
Unknown	16	<1
Subtotal	**3128**	
Not answered	25	
Grand Total	**3153**	

Just over half, 56.6% (1772/3128) of the patients were admitted via the emergency department (Table 3.2). The next largest group were patients admitted following referral or their GP or dental practitioner, (597/3128; 19%); and patients transferred in from another hospital (221/3128; 7.1%).

In the opinion of the advisors, 2058/2250, (91.5%) patients were admitted as an emergency, (Table 3.3).

Table 3.3 Emergency admission

Emergency admission	n	%
Yes	2058	91.5
No	192	8.5
Subtotal	**2250**	
Insufficient data	52	
Grand Total	**2302**	

Health status on admission

For each case included the clinician completing the questionnaire was asked to assess the health status of the patient (Table 3.4). Anaesthetists and surgeons will recognise this as the American Society of Anesthesiologists (ASA) score. All patients in this study died and therefore this defines their health status on admission.

Table 3.4 Health status on admission

Health status on admission	n	%
A normal healthy patient	52	1.7
A patient with mild systemic disease	244	8.0
A patient with severe systemic disease	743	24.2
A patient with incapacitating systemic disease	1368	44.6
A moribund patient	657	21.4
Subtotal	**3064**	
Not answered	89	
Grand Total	**3153**	

Of the patients in this sample 68.8% were admitted with a severe or incapacitating illness, (743/3064 and 1368/3064 respectively). Of the patients in this study 657 were moribund on admission. The 52 patients admitted as 'normal healthy patients' for example would represent a patient involved in an accident who had previously been systemically fit and healthy.

Overall quality of care

Figure 3.2 demonstrates that the quality of care received by two thirds (1337/2195; 60.9%) of patients in this study was judged, by the advisors, to be good practice. However, in 34.2% (750/2195) of patients there was room for improvement and in 4.9% (108/2195) of cases care was judged to have been less than satisfactory by the advisors. In 107 cases there was insufficient data to assess the case.

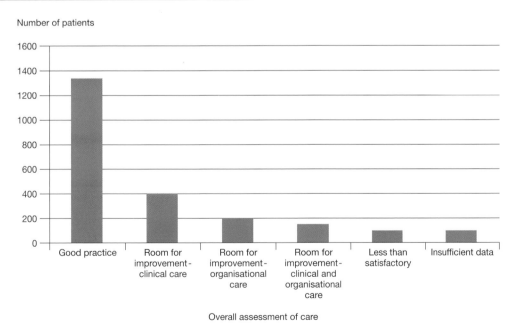

Figure 3.2 Overall assessment of care as judged by the advisors

4 - Process of care following admission

Excludes paediatrics		Denominator
Clinical questionnaire	Total population	3059
	Admitted under a surgeon	1354
	Admitted under a physician	1442
	Unable to determine admitting specialty	263
	Population who underwent a procedure or intervention	709
Assessment form	Total population	2225
	Underwent a procedure	474
	Did not undergo a procedure	1694
	Unable to determine	57
Clinical questionnaire cross referenced with the assessment form		2090

Good organisation of the admission process is the first step in ensuring that delay is minimised and that patients are seen and assessed by an appropriate health care professional in a timely manner and in an appropriate location. Since the publication of *'Functioning as a Team'* in 2002[1] and *'Emergency Admissions: A journey in the right direction?'* in 2007[3] there have been a number of changes in the working pattern of doctors, and the types of facilities into which patients are admitted. The increasing pressures of complying with the European Working Time Directive (EWTD), meeting government targets and the ever increasing move toward greater levels of sub-specialisation, might all be expected to have affected practice.

Although we have attempted to draw some comparisons with the findings from both the 2002 and 2007 reports, it is important to emphasise that direct comparisons were not possible. The 2002 report dealt with surgery and anaesthesia only, and included only those patients who underwent an operation. The 2007 report dealt with all emergency admissions, and not only included patients dying within seven days of admission, but also those transferred to critical care and those dying in the community within seven days of discharge.

Many of the findings within this current report are based upon the detailed analysis and peer review by the advisors, who have painstakingly scrutinised the clinical questionnaires and medical records provided. When interpreting these data it is important to recognise that the advisors were only able to form an impression based upon the information available to them. All too often they were frustrated by the missing information within the documentation.

Delay to admission

Table 4.1 shows that the incidence of cases where admission was judged by the advisors to be delayed was 5.5% (111/2014). There was judged to have been a slightly greater level of delay in admission, for those patients who ultimately underwent a procedure. However, the clinician completing the questionnaire believed that the delay in admission affected outcome in 1% (31/2921) of cases; it did not affect outcome in 2764 cases, was unknown in 126 and was not answered in 138 cases.

Delay between arrival and first assessment

From the clinical questionnaire it could be seen that the majority of patients (2038/2647;77%) had received an initial assessment within one hour (Figure 4.1). In 394 cases it was not possible to determine the time from admission to initial assessment.

Table 4.1 Delay in admission compared with patients who underwent a procedure

Admission delayed	Total population		Procedure		No procedure		Unspecified
	n	%	n	%	n	%	n
Yes	111	5.5	34	8	76	4.9	1
No	1903	94.5	389	92	1469	95.1	45
Subtotal	2014		423		1545		46
Insufficient data	211		51		149		11
Grand Total	2225		474		1694		57

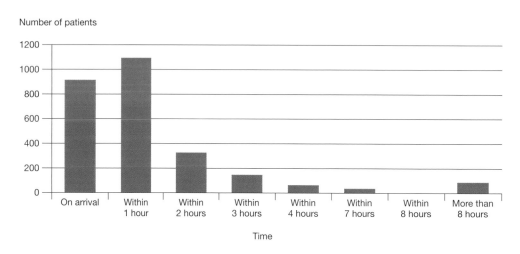

Figure 4.1 Time between arrival and initial assessment as assessed by self reporting from treating clinicians

When the same question was addressed by advisors using the data derived from the medical records, they were unable to determine the time to first assessment in 1172 cases. Where it could be determined the number of patients seen in less than one hour was 635/1053 (60.3%). Furthermore, the majority (1009/1053; 95.8%) of patients received an initial assessment within four hours of admission (Figure 4.2), and this may well be a consequence of the four hour emergency department waiting time target. Advisors questioned whether some of the initial assessments were being undertaken by junior trainees rather than a more senior doctor, in order to avoid breaching the four hour target[4].

Re-admissions

Table 4.2 overleaf shows that the percentage of patients in this study who had previously been discharged for the same condition was 4.5% (135/3021). The rate was higher for medical than surgical admissions, however where a procedure was undertaken (in this admission where the patient died) 4% (28/701) of those patients had been re-admitted. It is important to remember that all of these patients died within 96 hours of this admission, and therefore this does not reflect the overall reportable re-admission rate for Trusts.

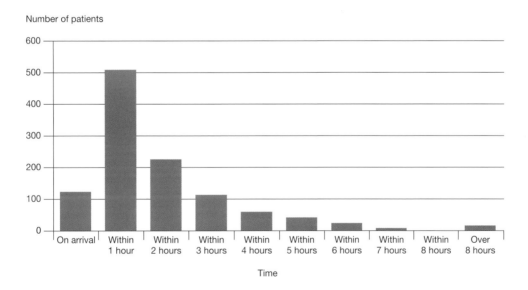

Number of patients

Time

Figure 4.2 Time between arrival and assessment as judged by advisors from case notes

Table 4.2 Re-admissions for a failed discharge

Re-admission	Total population		Admitted under a surgeon		Admitted under a physician		Underwent a procedure	
	n	%	n	%	n	%	n	%
Yes	135	4.5	50	3.7	71	5	28	4
No	2845	94.2	1277	95.2	1338	93.8	666	95
Unknown	41	1.4	14	1	18	1.3	7	1
Subtotal	3021		1341		1427		701	
Not answered	38		13		15		8	
Grand Total	3059		1354		1442		709	

Inappropriate admissions

In the opinion of the clinicians who completed the questionnaire, 4.3% (128/2981) of all admissions were unnecessary; this was not answered in 78 cases. The unnecessary admissions included eight patients undergoing a procedure. Of the128 patients admitted unnecessarily 112 patients were not expected to survive and it was the opinion of the clinician completing the questionnaire that they could have been managed in the community. These findings were similar to the findings of the 2007 report, where 5.9% of emergency admissions that resulted in death or transfer to critical care were judged to have been unnecessary.

Location of admission

Figure 4.3 illustrates to what type of location patients with different health status, on admission, were admitted. To surgeons and anaesthetists, the descriptors of health status will be recognisable as the American Society of Anesthesiologists (ASA) scoring system. However because physicians are not so familiar with this grading system, the textual descriptions only were used in this study. Interpretation of these data should be undertaken with caution, as it is recognised that when asked to judge the health status of the patient on admission, some clinicians may consider the status at various times after the initial admission which might explain the 'normal healthy patient' description.

There appeared to be very little difference in the way in which wards, specialist or critical care facilities were used, between surgeons and physicians. However, it appeared that patients described as moribund were more likely to be admitted to a general ward under the care of a surgeon, but more likely to go to a specialist ward if under the care of a physician. Given that 91.5% of the patients in this study were adimitted as an emergency, this may well reflect the difference in organisation of acute on call services for surgery and medicine.

When the assessment of overall care offered to ASA 3 and 4 patients by physicians and surgeons was compared, there was little difference observed in the quality of the care received.

Initial assessment

Previous groups of advisors have associated timely initial assessment by a clinician with sufficient experience with better quality of care. With respect to medicine the Royal College of Physicians has recommended that patients should be seen by a consultant within 12 hours of the initial assessment and in a shorter time period as appropriate[5].

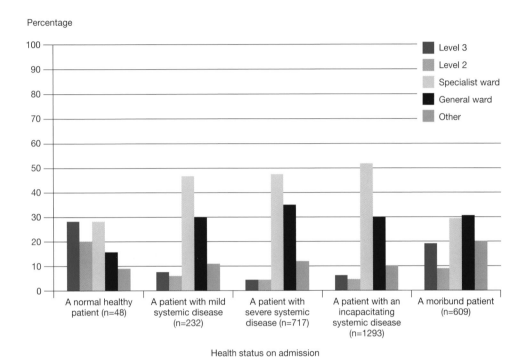

Percentage

Figure 4.3 Location of admission by health status on admission (total population)

There appeared to be a notable difference between the different surgical specialties, with regard to the seniority of clinician, who made the initial assessment (Figure 4.4 overleaf). In some of the smaller specialties, consultant involvement was high, although it should be noted that there were only small numbers of cases. In those larger specialties responsible for the majority of emergency and urgent admissions, a high percentage of patients were initially assessed by foundation year (FY)1-2/senior house officer (SHO) and house officer (HO) grades. Whilst it is to be expected in the larger specialties that many patients will be quite appropriately assessed initially by foundation doctors, it should be recalled that this sample is predominantly an elderly and sick group of patients admitted as emergencies, and in many of these patients there was considerable delay in consultant review, and furthermore the diagnosis was being made by foundation doctors. Specialist registrars (SpRs) undertook a large proportion of initial assessments in neurosurgery,

cardiothoracic and plastic surgery, but in the larger specialties SpRs were not so frequently involved in the initial assessment of patients. Advisors noted that the reduction in exposure of specialist trainees over time to the initial assessment of sick emergency patients might have a detrimental effect upon training.

As in previous studies, advisors noted the difficulty in identifying the grade of assessor. All professional groups who have issued guidance on good record keeping have stressed the importance of recording the seniority and specialty of the doctor undertaking assessment. This should include names, not just initials or signatures. The 2007 NCEPOD report recommended:

"The quality of medical note-keeping needs to improve. All entries in notes should be legible, contemporaneous and prompt. In addition, they should be legibly signed, dated and timed with a clear designation attached."[3]

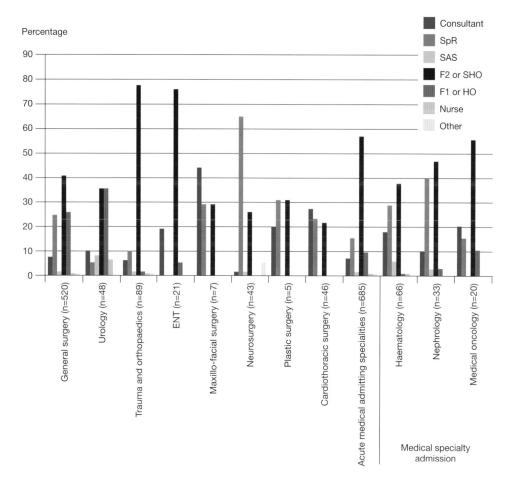

Percentage

Consultant
SpR
SAS
F2 or SHO
F1 or HO
Nurse
Other

General surgery (n=520)
Urology (n=48)
Trauma and orthopaedics (n=89)
ENT (n=21)
Maxillo-facial surgery (n=7)
Neurosurgery (n=43)
Plastic surgery (n=5)
Cardiothoracic surgery (n=46)
Acute medical admitting specialities (n=685)
Haematology (n=66)
Nephrology (n=33)
Medical oncology (n=20)

Medical specialty admission

Figure 4.4 Specialty and grade of first assessor

Location of initial assessment

The majority of patients in this sample were first assessed in the emergency department (Figure 4.5), however slightly more medical patients were first assessed in an assessment unit and more surgical patients were assessed on specialist wards. This may be explained by the finding of the 2007 report that whilst almost all acute hospitals had a medical assessment unit, only 60% had a surgical assessment unit.

Delays in first assessment

Advisors judged there to have been a delay in the first assessment in 4.6% (136/2987) cases, this could not be assessed in 72 cases. As in previous studies where delay in assessment occurred, the overall quality of care was more likely to be vulnerable to criticism (Figure 4.6).

Percentage

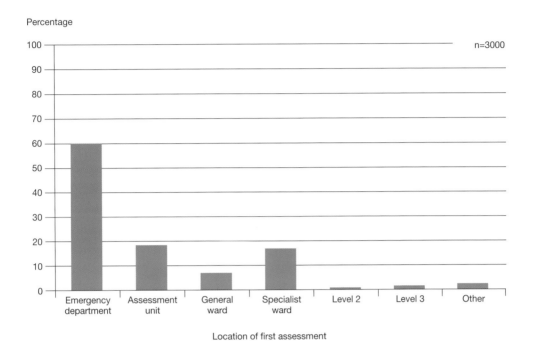

Figure 4.5 Location of first assessment

Percentage

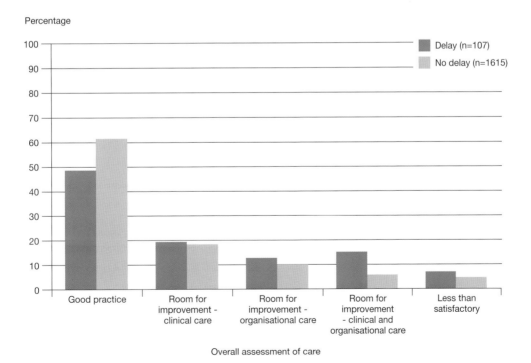

Figure 4.6 Overall assessment of care by delay in first review

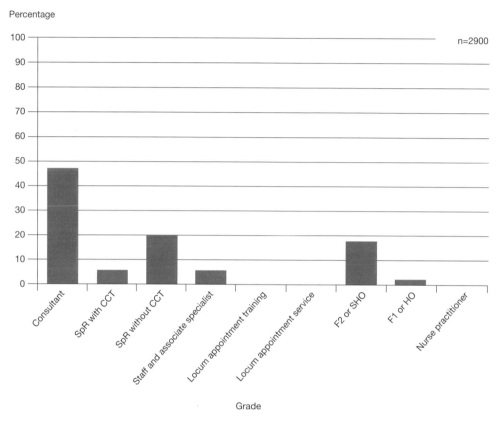

Percentage

n=2900

Grade

Figure 4.7 Grade of most senior healthcare professional making the diagnosis

Decision making

Consultant involvement
Consultants were involved in making the diagnosis in almost half of these patients, (1364/2900, 47%; not answered in 159 cases). However there were still a large number cases in which the diagnosis was made by FY doctors and HOs (581/2900, 20% - including HO and SHO) (Figure 4.7). There was no obvious difference in consultant input between those patients admitted under surgeons or physicians.

Consultants became less likely to be involved in making the diagnosis as the evening and night wore on. In the evening and at night time HOs, SHOs or FY doctors

were making the diagnosis in about 1 in 4 cases, (154/613; not answered in 40 cases) (Figure 4.8).

Time from admission to first consultant review

In this study approximately 70% (1502/2123; not answered in 936 cases) of patients were assessed by a consultant within 12 hours of admission and approximately 95% of patients were assessed within 24 hours (2023/2123). There was no discernible difference between the time taken for consultant review by surgeons or physicians. However this does not tell the whole story, as consultant review may be required in a much shorter time than these standards, where the condition of the patient requires it. In the view of the advisors, there was

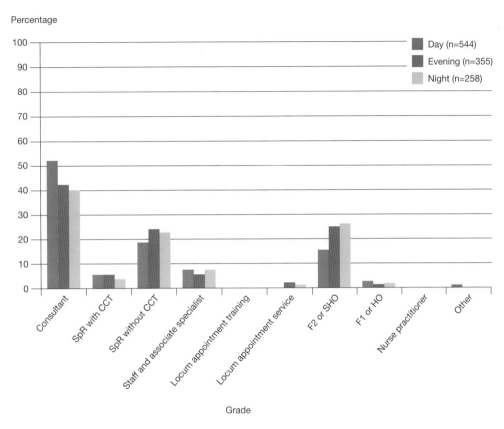

Percentage

Day (n=544)
Evening (n=355)
Night (n=258)

Grade

Figure 4.8 Grade of doctor making the diagnosis

a clinically important delay in consultant review in 24.9% (407/1635) of cases, (there was insufficient data to assess in 590 cases). As shown in Figure 4.9 overleaf, the median time between first review and first consultant review was substantially different according to whether patients were judged to have undergone a clinically significant delay. This possibly reflects the importance attached, by the advisors, to timely consultant review.

Management plan

Concern was expressed in the 2007 report, that documentation of a management plan was incomplete or absent in a number of cases.

In this study the advisors found no evidence of a documented management plan in 6.2% (130/2199) of cases, (insufficient data to assess in 115 cases). Advisors were of the opinion that given the fragmentation of clinical teams, and loss of the traditional "Firm" structure and the continuity of care associated with those structures, the documentation of a clear management plan within the medical records is an increasingly important priority.

Percentage

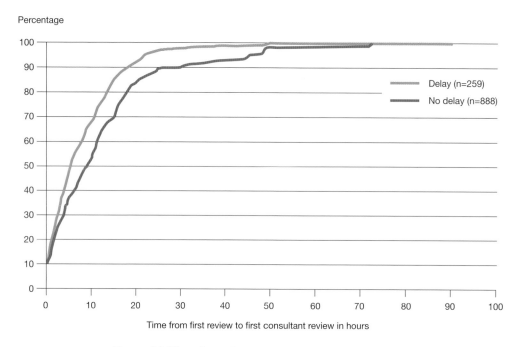

Time from first review to first consultant review in hours

**Figure 4.9 Time from first review to consultant review
by delay in consultant review**

Number of patients

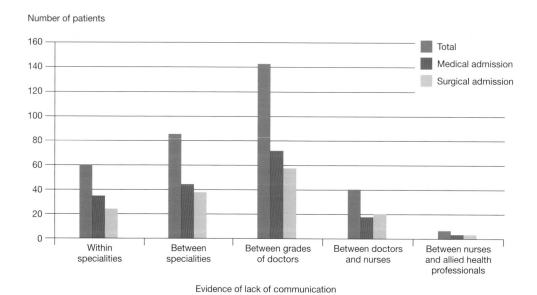

Evidence of lack of communication

Figure 4.10 Lack of team communication

Communication

Good documentation of clinical findings, clearly written management plans and robust systems for handover are all increasingly vital elements required to ensure that care is not jeopardised by poor communication. Communication is vital, not only between members of the same teams, but also between different professional groups, and where present, members of the hospital at night team. Advisors expressed concern that in a number of cases there was evidence of poor communication at all levels (Figure 4.10).

Overall the advisors identified lack of communication as an important issue in 13.5% of cases (267/1983) and there was insufficient data to assess in 107 cases. Due to the fact that this is a selected sample, this study may understate the true magnitude of the problem, as advisors are only able to make a judgement about deficiencies in communication where there was sufficient evidence from the records for them to do so with a reasonable degree of confidence. Similarly it is worth noting that this sample might well overestimate the problem too.

Figure 4.10 indicates that the problem with communication is not only horizontal, between different clinical teams and professional groups, but also vertically between different grades of staff within clinical teams. Advisors expressed concern that the modernisation of working patterns, including shift work, cross cover between clinical teams and the reduction in direct contact between trainees and consultants during the working week might all contribute to less efficient communication between those health care professionals involved in the care of a single patient.

A variety of different approaches are used to cover the hospital at night. Hospitals were asked in the organisational questionnaire whether they had a functioning Hospital at Night team. Of the hospital responses, 186/298 (62.4%) indicated that they had a Hospital at Night team. The composition and operation of these teams varied as shown in Table 4.3.

There was considerable reliance upon multi-professional multi-specialty cross cover arrangements. A co-ordinated handover of patients only occurred in 24.2% of these teams. The reliance upon multi-specialty cross cover, combined with the lack of dedicated time for co-ordinated handover is likely to be an important factor in poor communications which have been identified. It also means that patients are less likely to receive timely care from clinicians with the appropriate skills and knowledge.

Table 4.3 Hospital at Night cover

Type of cover	n	%
Multi-professional team	57	30.6
Multi-professional team and co-ordinated handover	13	7
Multi-professional team, co-ordinated bleep and multi-specialty cross cover	56	30.1
Multi-professional team and multi-specialty cross cover	5	2.7
Co-ordinated handover	45	24.2
Co-ordinated handover and multi-specialty cross cover	1	<1
Multi-specialty cross cover	9	4.8
Subtotal	**186**	
Not answered	111	
Grand Total	**297**	

29

Key findings

Consultant involvement in assessment and diagnosis becomes less frequent in the evenings and at night time, when the diagnosis was made to be made by foundation doctors and SHOs in 25% (154/613) of cases. In some specialties this may be appropriate, but many of these emergency patients had complex conditions requiring urgent senior input.

In 25% (407/1635) of cases there was, in the view of the advisors, a clinically important delay in the first review by a consultant.

Poor communication between and within clinical teams was identified by the advisors as an important issue in 13.5% (267/1983) of cases.

Poor documentation remains commonplace. This hinders effective communication between team members and makes the subsequent assessment and audit of care difficult.

Recommendations

The seniority of clinical staff assessing a patient and making a diagnosis should be determined by the clinical needs of the patient, and not the time of day. Services should be organised to ensure that patients have access to consultants whenever they are required. The organisation of services will vary from specialty to specialty, but may require input from clinical directors, medical directors and the Strategic Health Authority.

Better systems of handover must be established, and this must include high quality legible medical record keeping. (Consultants)

The benefits and risks to patient safety of reduced working hours should be fully assessed, and clinical teams must be organised to ensure that there is continuity of care. (Clinical Directors)

5 - Surgery and anaesthesia

Excludes paediatrics		Denominator
Clinical questionnaire	Total population	3059
	Admitted under a surgeon	1354
	Underwent a procedure	709
Assessment form	Total population	2225
Organisational questionnaire		297

Unlike the previous 2002 NCEPOD study, which only examined the care of surgical patients who died following an operation, this study included patients who died following admission under the care of a surgeon, but who did not undergo an operation.

Demographic data

Based on the returned clinical questionnaire 709 patients included in the study underwent either a surgical or medical procedure.

NCEPOD classifies the urgency of a procedure by the following grades:

Immediate - Immediate life or limb saving. Resuscitation simultaneous with surgical/interventional treatment.
Urgent - Acute onset or deterioration of conditions that threaten life, limb or organ survival; fixation of fractures; relief of distressing symptoms including acute surgical admissions not requiring an operation.
Expedited - Stable patient requiring early intervention for a condition that is not an immediate threat to life, limb or organ.
Elective - Surgical/interventional procedure planned or booked in advance of routine admission to hospital.

For those patients undergoing a procedure, Figure 5.1 shows the urgency using the NCEPOD classification.

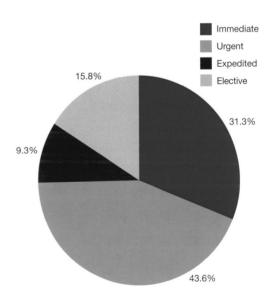

Figure 5.1 Classification of urgency of intervention

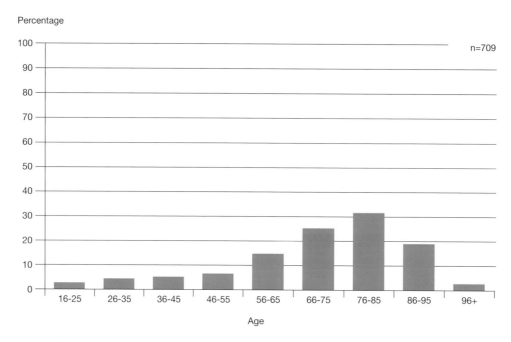

Percentage

n=709

Age

Figure 5.2 Age profile of the patients who underwent a surgical procedure

As with the total sample in this study the gender split was roughly equal with 49.1% of the patients male and 50.9% female (Table 5.1), and the sample was mainly over the age of 55 (Figure 5.2).

Table 5.1 Gender of patients who underwent a procedure

Gender	n	%
Male	348	49.1
Female	361	50.9
Grand Total	**709**	

The physical status of the patient as defined by the ASA grading relating to the NCEPOD classification is shown in Figure 5.3.

Those patients in the ASA1 and elective groups were reviewed. Causes of death were all recognised complications of the surgical procedures undertaken.

When considering the patients from this dataset who underwent a surgical procedure the proportion of patients undergoing surgery under different specialties has changed little from the 2002 report[1]. However what these data show was that a proportion of patients were admitted under a surgical specialty and died without undergoing surgery (Table 5.2). This was particularly notable for general surgery.

Number of patients

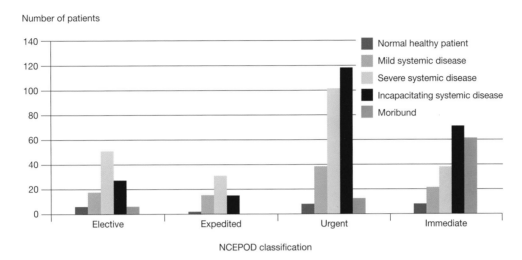

NCEPOD classification

**Figure 5.3 Physical status of the patient as defined by the
ASA grading and urgency of procedure**

Table 5.2 Surgical specialty at the time of admission

	2006/07						2000/01		1994/5
	Admitted under the care of a surgeon		Admitted under the care of a surgeon and underwent a procedure		Admitted under the care of a surgeon at the time of procedure and underwent a procedure		Underwent a procedure		Underwent a procedure
Surgery specialty at admission and operation	n	%	n	%	n	%	n	%	%
General surgery (including vascular)	762	62.2	210	47.2	233	51.4	1044	49	52
Orthopaedic	228	18.6	116	26.1	102	22.5	562	27	23
Cardiothoracic	50	4.1	44	9.9	49	10.8	123	6	6
Urology	68	5.5	19	4.3	14	3.1	121	6	6
Neurosurgery	45	3.7	28	6.3	33	7.3	83	4	4
Paediatric	2	0.2	2	0.4	3	0.7	48	2	NA
Gynaecology	27	2.2	11	2.5	7	1.5	45	2	5
Otorhinolaryngology	26	2.1	9	2.0	6	1.3	44	2	1
Plastic surgery	9	0.7	3	0.7	3	0.7	19	<1	1
Opthalmology	0	0.0	0	0.0	0	0.0	16	<1	1
Oral/maxillofacial	9	0.7	3	0.7	3	0.7	9	<1	<1
Subtotal	**1226**		**445**		**453**				
Accidental and Emergency or other	138		21		1				
Grand Total	**1364**		**466**		**454**		**2114**		

NCEPOD has in the past identified a number of cases, where in retrospect, futile operations were performed, when non-surgical palliative management would have been more appropriate. Similarly, the advisors noted in this study, that there were cases where, for a variety of reasons, an operation from which the patient might potentially have benefited was not performed.

Case study 1

A teenage patient became neutropenic following chemotherapy for a sarcoma. The patient was admitted under the general paediatricians, unwell and with soft tissue infection over the chest wall. A paediatric specialist registrar diagnosed cellulitis. The patient was reviewed by a surgical specialist registrar who raised the possibility of necrotising fasciitis. There was no senior surgical input and no action was taken. The patient deteriorated over the next 12 hours and died without further surgical review or intervention.

Un-operated necrotising fasciitis is fatal. In the view of the advisors early consultant review and active treatment might have prevented the death of this patient.

Case study 2

A teenager was involved in a road traffic accident. On admission they had a Glasgow Coma Score (GCS) of 14/15. A CT scan demonstrated a subdural haematoma. An emergency department specialist registrar discussed the patient with a neurosurgical SpR and a further CT was ordered. Transfer was not accepted despite deterioration in the patient's GCS to 12/15 over the next two hours. Following a further deterioration over another hour to GCS 8/15 the patient was intubated and following further discussion with a neurosurgical specialist registrar a third CT scan was ordered. During the scan the patient's endotracheal tube became blocked and the patient became hypoxic which lead to raised intracranial pressure. Thirty six hours later the patient was declared brain dead and ventilation withdrawn.

The advisors questioned whether with senior involvement at an earlier stage, clear diagnosis and a decisive management plan, could this patient have undergone craniotomy and potentially avoided this outcome? Was this a case of over-enthusiastic "gate keeping" to protect scarce neurosurgical resources?

Percentage

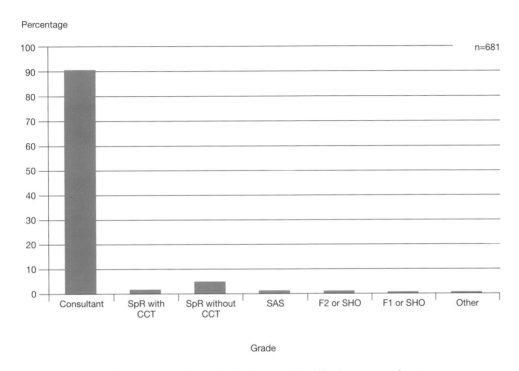

Figure 5.4 Grade of clinician consulted before procedure

Some surgery was undertaken in patients who were not expected to survive. In this study these were most commonly: laparotomy (19), craniotomy (5) and operations for fractured neck of femur (4). Advisors recognised that in many cases they did not have sufficient information to enable them to make retrospective judgments about the actual decision taken, however they noted that in a small number of cases, decisions were taken involving sick and complex patients by junior trainees without consultation with consultants (Figure 5.4).

The proportion of cases in which a consultant was consulted before a procedure was undertaken had changed little from the 93% given in the 2002 report.

Consent

The majority 91.7% (1995/2175) of the patients admitted in this study were emergency or urgent admissions (insufficient data in 50 cases). Therefore the majority of procedures were performed on an immediate or urgent basis. Although the NCEPOD classification changed in the time between the 2002 report and the present study, the degree of urgency of operation can still be compared, and there was little change in the proportion of immediate and urgent cases (74.8%, 474/633 in this study against 75% in 2002), (not answered in 76 cases).

Some of these patients did not have evidence of a formal consent form retained in the clinical records. However, where consent was taken in emergency cases, very junior foundation doctors and house officers were more likely to be involved (Figure 5.5). Whilst this does not necessarily indicate poor practice, advisors raised the issue that in a number of very complex cases the junior trainees would not have had sufficient knowledge to be able to give, and interpret, the information required for patients to make meaningful choices and give valid consent.

Interpretation of these data also requires caution. Documentation was poor, and it may be that a senior clinician undertook a thorough discussion with the patient and or relatives, and that the consent form was simply completed by a junior member of the team to document that the consent process had been completed. Whilst there is no absolute legal requirement for documentary evidence to record the material details of the discussions which formed the basis of the consent, there are strong recommendations from all professional bodies, the Department of Health, and the professional indemnity organisations that there should be a written record of the consent, or reasons why consent was not obtained. Where there is disagreement between patient and doctor about what was said and in the absence of any contemporaneous written record the courts sometimes prefer the version of events provided by the patient to that of the doctor.

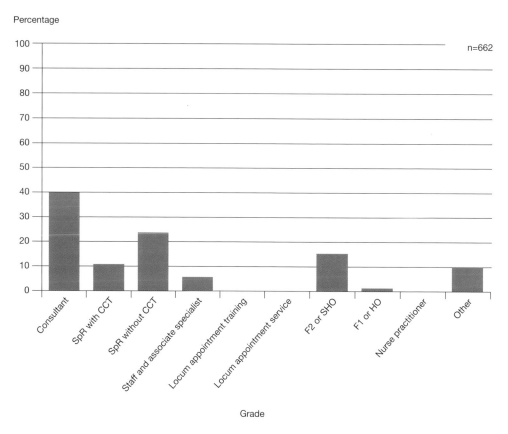

Figure 5.5 Grade of clinician taking consent

Delays between admission and operation

Delays occurred in 13.8% (85/617) of those cases undergoing a procedure (not answered in 92 cases). Where reasons for the delay were given, these included: lack of sufficient theatre time, delay in consultant review, delay by junior doctors in reaching the correct diagnosis, delay in recognising the need for surgery because of a failure to recognise the seriousness of the patient's condition and to seek appropriate senior advice.

Availability of theatres, recovery, and staff for emergency surgery

In this study 129/148 (87%) of hospitals (who admitted surgical patients) had dedicated emergency (NCEPOD) theatre lists available (not answered in 1 case). Of these just under 2/3 (Monday to Wednesday 86/148; Thursday and Friday 87/148; Saturday and Sunday 94/148) were available 24 hours 7 days per week. At units where patients were admitted under a trauma and orthopaedic surgeon during the study period, 83/84 (99%) of hospitals had dedicated trauma lists of which only 31% (26/84) were available 24 hours 7 days per week; this figure increased to (71%) 60/84 available 7 days a week, (though not 24 hours). In 6/143 (4.2%) hospitals where patients were admitted under a surgical specialty during the study period, there was no dedicated consultant anaesthetist rostered to cover the emergency or trauma theatres, (not answered in 6 cases). In 1/145 unit admitting patients under a surgical specialty, there was no staffed recovery area for emergency surgery; In 122/145 (83%) staffed recovery facilities were available 24 hours/day 7 days per week (not answered in 2 cases). Dedicated recovery staff were available in 106/147 (72%) hospitals, but in many cases, recovery for emergency patients was provided by theatre staff and/or the anaesthetist (34/147, 23%), (not answered in 2 cases) NCEPOD has previously highlighted the fact that reliance upon the theatre staff and anaesthetists for recovery of the patient can lead to delays for other emergency patients, and does not make the most efficient use of staffed emergency theatres.

There were still many hospitals without access to fully staffed emergency theatres 24 hours/day 7 days per week. Whilst it is of note that the number of inappropriate operations conducted late at night by junior staff had reduced since first highlighted by NCEPOD, this does not mean that hospitals can dispense with emergency theatres. These must still be available without delay for those patients with life or limb threatening emergencies, requiring immediate surgical intervention.

Prioritisation

Table 5.3 Clinical priority grading system

Priority grading system	n	%
Yes	95	66.9
No	42	29.6
Unknown	5	3.5
Subtotal	**142**	
Not answered	7	
Grand Total	**149**	

As the data in Table 5.3 show, 66.9% (95/142) of the acute hospitals (who admitted a patient under a surgical specialty during the study period) have a clinical grading system for determining clinical priority in emergency surgery. Of those that did, 48 sites specified the use of the NCEPOD grading system. Operating list order was recorded as being commonly determined between surgeons and anaesthetists.

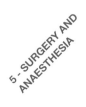

Treatment intention

In a number of cases the purpose of the procedure was unclear.

Table 5.4 Purpose of procedure

Purpose of procedure	n	%
Diagnostic	80	13.2
Diagnostic & curative	29	4.8
Diagnostic & curative & palliative	1	<1
Diagnostic & palliative	7	1.2
Curative	388	63.9
Curative & palliative	4	<1
Palliative	98	16.1
Subtotal	**607**	
Not answered	102	
Grand Total	**709**	

In one case a procedure was reported to have been undertaken with diagnostic, curative and palliative intent (Table 5.4). Whilst the purpose of surgery may change, as unexpected findings emerge, all reasonable steps should be taken to ensure that patients are not subjected to unnecessary and futile procedures, because of lack of careful pre-operative assessment, and multi-disciplinary team involvement. In a number of cases there appeared to be confusion about whether procedures were being undertaken with palliative of curative intent.

It should be noted that the World Health Organisation defines palliative care as follows:

"Palliative care is an approach that improves the quality of life of patients and their families facing the problem associated with life-threatening illness, through the prevention and relief of suffering by means of early identification and impeccable assessment and treatment of pain and other problems, physical, psychosocial and spiritual. Palliative care:
- *provides relief from pain and other distressing symptoms;*
- *affirms life and regards dying as a normal process;*
- *intends neither to hasten or postpone death;"*[6]

Prior to undertaking surgery, there should be a clear management plan, and in complex cases, where time permits, decision making, including determination of the treatment intent, should be done by an appropriate multi-disciplinary team, with the patient and carers fully informed and involved in the decision making process.

Health care professionals in theatre

The majority of surgical admissions were classed as emergency or urgent and operations undertaken were on an immediate or urgent basis. Advisors noted the relative infrequency with which specialist registrars were present in theatre (Figure 5.6). There now appears to be a shift away from trainees operating on emergencies without a consultant present, to consultants operating without any trainees present. Whilst it is true that the medical notes including the operation note are often poorly completed and may not record all those present or even assisting in theatre, it is more likely that the clinician completing the questionnaire will recall the individuals who were present and assisting in theatre for those patients who died. This raises the question whether surgical trainees are getting sufficient exposure and training in the management of surgical emergencies. It is important to draw the distinction here between the undesirable practice of junior trainees operating alone out of hours, and beyond their own level of competence, and the desirable practice of trainees operating under appropriate supervision in order to gain exposure and experience in the management of the emergency surgical patient.

Number of patients

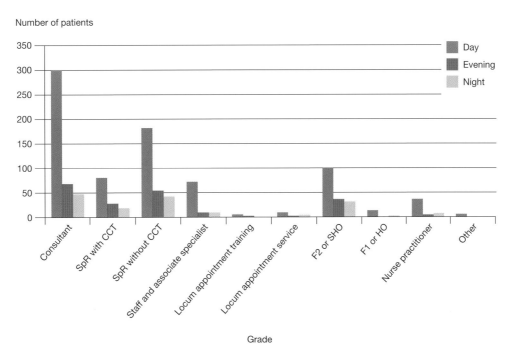

Figure 5.6 Grade of health care professionals in theatre by time of day

Additional consideration was given to the level of supervision of trainees in theatres, when they are operating. Whilst the majority of operations were performed by consultants (61%, 361/591), 28% (166/591) were performed by SpRs (other grades = 64; not answered in 118 cases).

Where the most senior operating surgeon was not a consultant, the trainee was operating without a consultant scrubbed in theatre in the majority of cases, albeit, the consultant was present in either the operating suite or elsewhere in the hospital in most cases (Table 5.5).

Table 5.5 Levels of supervision when the most senior operating clinician was not a consultant.

Level of supervision	n	%
Supervised scrubbed	24	12.2
Unsupervised in theatre/procedural room	49	25.0
Unsupervised in hospital	85	43.4
Other	38	19.4
Subtotal	**196**	
Not answered	37	
Grand Total	**233**	

These data suggest that in this sample not only were trainees less frequently in theatres, but when they were, they were not receiving direct supervision at the operating table. This raised concerns, that trainees are not getting quality training in emergency surgery. It also raises the question about the levels of assistance available for consultants operating without any trainees in theatre. There is still inconsistency in the nomenclature and classification of levels of supervision between different specialties, using different log books. There needs to be a cross specialty consensus to achieve a consistent approach to the classification of levels of clinical supervision.

There is a great deal of debate about the implications of implementation of the European Working Time Directive (EWTD) on continuity of care, patient safety versus training and fatigue considerations. The Government expressed the opinion that the balance is in favour of 48 hours[7], while at least one Royal College is of the view that somewhere closer to 65 hours is a more appropriate balance[8]. There is likely to be a crossing point at which the benefits of continuity of care derived from working longer hours, becomes overridden by the dangers of fatigue. Ideally well conducted research should be undertaken to ascertain where that cross-over point is. It is likely that there is no one ideal figure which is optimal for all specialties, and for all individuals, however unless there is evidence underpinning a political will to challenge the EWTD through the European Parliament, other mechanisms must be developed in order to address the lack of continuity of out of hours care, and the availability of appropriately trained staff 24 hours per day. A number of models have been suggested, and these include the separation of emergency from elective care, and greater centralisation of specialist services. These need to be balanced with geographical access considerations[9,10].

Peri-operative complications

In the view of the advisors 257/433 patients experienced a peri-operative complication prior to death (insufficient data to assess in 41 cases). Of these complications 42/173 were judged by the advisors to be avoidable (insufficient data to assess in 84 cases). The majority of peri-operative complications were judged to have had an adverse effect on outcome (211/223, insufficient data in 34 cases). In these patients who died complications did not occur more frequently when the operation was undertaken in evenings or at night.

Examples of avoidable complications included, misplaced endotracheal tube, aspiration, inadequate management of intra-operative hypotension, inappropriate method of central line insertion, failure to give appropriate prophylaxis for deep vein thrombosis, and failure to send the patient to the appropriate level of post operative critical care.

Surgical case studies

Throughout this study, advisors undertaking the peer review of cases identified a number of recurring themes:
- poor communication and team working;
- lack of multidisciplinary care;
- poor end of life care planning;
- lack of involvement of palliative care teams;
- inadequate consent;
- deficiencies in diagnosis;
- delay in assessment and treatment;
- poor fluid and electrolyte management;
- failure to recognise or manage malnourishment;
- poor documentation;
- failure to adapt level of care to health status of the patient;
- failure of audit and critical incident reporting;
- neglect of deep vein thrombosis and antibiotic prophylaxis.

Many of the deficiencies identified were common to the various surgical specialties. To illustrate some of these, a number of case studies follow, drawn from several different surgical specialties.

Case study 3: general surgery

An elderly ASA 3 patient was re-admitted under general surgeons from a residential home. The patient had recently been discharged from a different team following care for abdominal pain associated with known diverticular disease; this had been resolved with conservative management. On this admission the patient complained of similar right hypochondrial pain and tenderness with a temperature of 38.5°C. Overnight the patient became hypotensive and was given 2 litres of intravenous fluids, but no antibiotics. At 09:00 the next day on the consultant ward round a diagnosis of peritonitis was established and arrangements were made to take patient to theatre for laparotomy. However, before a theatre became available the patient suffered a gastrointestinal bleed and died.

The advisors noted that the autopsy showed perforated diverticular disease and questioned whether there should have been a senior review earlier and whether the patient should have been given intravenous antibiotics?

Case study 4: vascular surgery

An elderly ASA 3 patient presented with an ischaemic leg at 17:30 on a Friday evening. The patient was admitted to a general surgical ward by a surgical senior house officer, who made arrangements for further investigations to be undertaken after the weekend. There was no evidence of any documented handover, and over the weekend there were no further entries in the medical records by medical staff. The nursing records indicated that the patient's condition was deteriorating. The leg ischaemia was worsened and the patient developed difficulty breathing. A series of different junior doctors saw the patient. Large volumes of intravenous saline were prescribed. No anticoagulants were prescribed. No early warning scoring was recorded, and the patient was not seen by either a physician or critical care outreach team. The first consultant input documented was on a surgical ward round at 10:00 the following Monday. An urgent critical care opinion was sought, but the patient arrested and died before this was undertaken.

The advisors judged that there had been a lack of senior input, there had been delay by junior staff in recognising the seriousness of the condition and that there was poor communication between the different staff looking after the patient. In addition to the communication issues, the fluid management was poor.

Case study 5: orthopaedics

An elderly patient was returned to a general surgical ward following hemi-arthroplasty for a fractured neck of femur. In the immediate postoperative period 10 litres of intravenous saline were administered over 12 hours. There was no senior input to care, which was managed by an orthopaedic senior house officer who did not seek any advice. No urinary catheter had been placed and the fluid balance charts were poorly completed. The patient died 20 hours postoperatively. The cause of death given on the death certificate was "cardiac failure".

The advisors considered it inappropriate for this patient to have been sent directly to a general surgery ward. The patient would have benefited from a greater degree of senior input and interdisciplinary care with medicine for the elderly.

Case study 6: cardiothoracic surgery

A middle aged patient presented with an acute dissection of the thoracic aorta. Discussion took place between a cardiothoracic and a cardiology specialist registrar without direct consultant input. A decision was taken to deny surgery but admit to a coronary care unit for medical management despite the fact that any prospect of survival without surgery was remote and despite the fact that there were no particular comorbidities to contra-indicate surgery. The patient deteriorated over the next 12 hours with more pain despite reasonable blood pressure control. There was no re-referral to the surgeons. The patient had a cardiac arrest and died.

The advisors questioned whether there was optimal team working between cardiology and cardiothoracic surgery and stated that there should have been involvement by consultants in the decision making process.

Case study 7: urology

An elderly patient was admitted on a planned basis for a transurethral resection of a bladder tumour. The patient was noted to have chest pains, a systolic heart murmur and was anaemic with haemoglobin of 9.7 g/dl. A previous admission had been cancelled, and an echocardiogram had been organised. This had demonstrated aortic stenosis. The only medication on admission was thyroxine. The patient had not attended for pre-anaesthetic assessment nor had their treatment been discussed at a multidisciplinary team meeting, and no cardiology opinion had been sought. The operation was performed under a spinal anaesthetic and the patient was hypotensive throughout the procedure (100/45). During the procedure, the bladder was perforated, although the surgeon completing the questionnaire indicated that there were no intra-operative problems. A pre-registration house officer (PRHO) was called to see the patient at 05:00 the following morning, because of worsening chest pain. There was no intavenous access and the

blood pressure was noted to be 65/35.Some ECG changes were noted. The blood pressure remained low, and the next evening the haemoglobin had dropped to 6.0 g/dl. Without any senior review, the PRHO ordered 3 units of blood, and this was given between 23:00 and 05:00 the following day. The patient was eventually seen at 08:00 on the 2nd postoperative day by a medical specialist registrar, who diagnosed a myocardial infarct with left ventricular failure and transferred the patient to the coronary care unit, where the patient arrested and died two hours later.

A PRHO should not have been managing this patient without senior input and the advisors noted that the PRHO failed to recognise the seriousness of the situation, and communication at all levels was poor. They considered whether a cardiologist should have been involved from the outset.

Case study 8: ear, nose and throat

A middle aged patient was re-admitted with skin breakdown three weeks after undergoing a radical neck dissection and pectoralis major flap for a squamous cell carcinoma of an unknown primary. The patient was known to abuse alcohol, and had had a previous history of peptic ulceration. The patient underwent a split skin graft to the neck wound, however in the immediate postoperative period they collapsed and passed a significant melaena. The patient had hypotension, a tachycardia, and haemoglobin was 6.4 g/dl. The ear, nose and throat senior house officer contacted the locum medical registrar. After a delay of six hours, the medical

registrar saw the patient and referred to the locum surgical specialist registrar. After a further delay of four hours, during which time the patient remained hypotensive, the patient arrested and died.

The advisors questioned whether there should have been better multi-disciplinary pre-operative preparation, including gastric protection and more senior involvement at an earlier stage. Advisors were concerned about the poor documentation and the lack of communication both within and between the different clinical teams involved in this patient's care.

Case study 9: gynaecology

A young patient was admitted for the elective hysteroscopic removal of a fibroid and dye test. There was no known pre-operative comorbidity and she was ASA 1 (a normal healthy patient). The surgery was uneventful however during the anaesthetic the patient became hypotensive, bradycardic and developed massive pulmonary oedema. Cardiopulmonary resuscitation was unsuccessful. The case was reported to the coroner and an autopsy undertaken. A cause of death could not be ascertained. The coroner's autopsy report commented upon the illegibility and incompleteness of the hospital records.

The advisors found no evidence to suggest that there had been any deficiency in the standard of care. However as with the coroner they noted that the record keeping was very poor.

These case studies drawn from each specialty illustrate the presentation of the recurring themes of remediable factors, identified throughout the study, and placed in the context of each specialty. Some of the generic issues require actions at Strategic Health Authority, and Trust level, particularly where re-configurations are required. Others require remediable action, which is specific to the individual specialties. Each specialty may have much to gain by reflecting upon how others tackle similar problems.

Organisational data

Decontamination

Table 5.6 Availability of decontamination facilities

Decontamination facilities available	n	%
On site	200	70.9
Off site	80	28.4
Unknown	2	<1
Subtotal	**282**	
Not answered	15	
Grand Total	**297**	

As the data in Table 5.6 shows, almost a third of sites had off site decontamination facilities. Furthermore, where decontamination facilities were only available off site, there were more likely to be operational problems in the service (28/78; 2 not answered), in comparison to sites where decontamination facilities are available on site, (39/197; 3 not answered). Examples of problems cited by clinicians included: postponement and delay of operations, prolonged anaesthetic times, whilst replacement instruments were located, and technical difficulties undertaking operations because substitute instruments had to be used.

Key findings

There was lack of involvement of trainees in emergency surgery in a supervised learning environment.

There was a lack of communication both between different grades of doctors within clinical teams, and between different clinical teams and other health care professionals.

There was a poor standard of record keeping. Good legible records, and coordinated handovers are essential if good communication between team members is to be established.

There were instances of poor decision making and lack of senior input, particularly in the evenings and night time.

Some of the basic aspects of clinical care continue to be neglected. In particular the monitoring, recording and management of fluid balance in the elderly and those with multiple comorbidities.

Recommendations

Systems of communication between doctors and other health care professionals must improve. In particular trainees must seek consultant input at an early stage to assist in the management of emergency patients. (Clinical Directors and Medical Directors)

The training of nurses and doctors must place emphasis on the basic skills of monitoring vital functions, recognising deterioration, and acting appropriately (which will often be to seek senior input). (Deaneries, Clinical Directors)

All trainees need to be exposed in an appropriate learning environment to the management of emergency patients. Clinical services must be organised to allow appropriately supervised trainee involvement. Organisation of services must address training needs, and this will vary from specialty to specialty. (Clinical Directors)

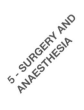

Anaesthesia

Excludes paediatrics		Denominator
Anaesthetic questionnaire	Total population	345
Assessment form	Underwent a procedure	474
Anaesthetic questionnaire by assessment form		235

This section of the report concerns the anaesthetic management of those patients who underwent a surgical procedure prior to death. The patient pathway from pre-operative assessment and consent through to postoperative recovery.

Pre-operative assessment (pre-admission)

Proper pre-operative assessment and record keeping is essential for good anaesthetic practice[11]. Before undergoing an operation that requires general or regional anaesthesia, provided by an anaesthetist, all patients must be seen by an anaesthetist (Table 5.7). The Association of Anaesthetists of Great Britain and Ireland recommend that:

"All patients must be seen by an anaesthetist before undergoing an operation that requires the services of an anaesthetist."[12].

Table 5.7 Evidence of pre-operative anaesthetic assessment

Evidence of pre-operative anaesthetic assessment	n	%
Yes	130	31.2
No	234	56.1
Unknown	53	12.7
Subtotal	417	
Not answered	57	
Grand Total	474	

There was evidence of pre-admission anaesthetic assessment in 31.2% (130/417) of patients in this group which might simply reflect the fact that this sample contained a high proportion of emergency admissions.

Evidence of pre-admission anaesthetic assessment was assessed against the urgency of the procedure undertaken. The number of patients seen by anaesthetists prior to admission was lower for immediate procedures (19/69) (insufficient data to assess in 9 cases) than for the other three categories (37/81 for urgent cases (insufficient data to assess in 10 cases), 7/17 for expedited (insufficient data to assess in 2 cases) and 15/33 for elective cases (insufficient data to assess in 9 cases). In a further five cases the urgency of the operation was not indicated.

It can be seen from Table 5.8 that pre-operative anaesthetic review, following admission to hospital, was documented in 68.8% (285/414) of cases. The disparity in these figures is likely to relate to the high proportion of urgent and immediate operations in this data set, equally the unavailability of some anaesthetic charts did not allow this fact to be verified.

Table 5.8 Documented anaesthetic review (pre-operative)

Documented pre-operative anaesthetic review	n	%
Yes	285	68.8
No	48	11.6
Unable to answer	81	19.6
Subtotal	414	
Not answered	60	
Grand Total	474	

It is possible that patients were seen by clinicians, but it had not been clearly documented. It is recommended that all anaesthetists document the time and date of their pre-operative visit and assessment[13].

Reasons why patients were not assessed by anaesthetists prior to surgery included:
- patient rushed to theatre;
- patient collapsed in anaesthetic room;
- surgery and cardio-pulmonary resuscitation at same time;
- transfer from another hospital with ruptured abdominal aortic aneurysm;
- transfer straight to theatre from another hospital.

Evidence of pre-operative anaesthetic information provided to the patient

It is well recognised that good pre-operative information affects a patient's ability to cope with stressful hospital admissions[14,15].

There was evidence of pre-operative anaesthetic information being given to patients in 128/227 (56.4%) patients (Table 5.9). The information may have been written or verbal during the pre-operative visit. Documentation of either written or verbal communication would aid confirming the validity of consent. In these cases where patients are extremely unwell it may reflect the competence of the patient in the immediate pre-

Table 5.9 Anaesthetic information provided to the patient – advisors' view

Anaesthetic information provided	n	%
Yes	128	56.4
No	99	43.6
Subtotal	227	
Insufficient data	247	
Grand Total	474	

operative period. However, it was not possible for the advisors to assess whether anaesthetic information had been provided in 183 cases.

Anaesthetic consent

A separate formal consent form signed by the patient for an anaesthetic is not required[16] and here the anaesthetist was only involved in obtaining consent in 60.4% (206/341) of procedures (Table 5.10). The decision to operate was however considered appropriate by the anaesthetists completing questionnaires in 97.5% (306/314) of cases, (not answered in 31 cases).

Table 5.10 Consent for anaesthesia was obtained by an anaesthetist

Consent for anaesthesia obtained by an anaesthetist	n	%
Yes	206	60.4
No	99	29.0
Unknown	36	10.6
Subtotal	341	
Not answered	5	
Grand Total	346	

It is recommended that a record of the consent to anaesthesia be recorded and by whom this consent is gained[16].

Comorbidities

The common comorbidities that patients presented with are shown in Table 5.11.

Table 5.11 Comorbidities that patients' presented with (answers may be multiple)

Comorbidities	n
Insulin dependent diabetes	15
Renal disease	70
Hypertension	160
Cardiac disease	183
Respiratory disease	85
Other	130

The advisors were of the opinion that in 91.5% (280/306) of cases the comorbidities detailed in Table 5.11 were managed adequately, (insufficient data in 8 cases). In 17.4% (58/334) of patients, clinicians completing the anaesthetic questionnaire indicated there was a delay in operating in order to optimise the patient's comorbidities (not answered in 11 cases).

Adequate optimisation of condition

Patients were considered by the advisors to be adequately prepared in 87.7% (278/317) of cases (Table 5.12). The commonest reasons for not being optimised that the advisors highlighted were investigation of cardiovascular status and fluid balance problems, insertion of central venous line, delay in surgery and lack of an intensive care bed.

Table 5.12 Adequate pre-operative optimisation of the patients' condition

Adequate pre-operative optimisation of the patients' condition	n	%
Yes	278	87.7
No	39	12.3
Subtotal	317	
Unable to answer	96	
Not answered	61	
Grand Total	474	

Appropriate grade of anaesthetist

The advisors were of the opinion that an appropriate grade of anaesthetist looked after the patient in 95.8% (206/215) of cases. However, it is important to note that the advisors were unable to assess this in 259/474 cases (Table 5.13).

Table 5.13 Appropriate grade of anaesthetist – advisors' view

Appropriate grade of anaesthetist	n	%
Yes	206	95.8
No	9	5.5
Subtotal	215	
Unable to answer	192	
Not answered	67	
Grand Total	474	

Number of patients

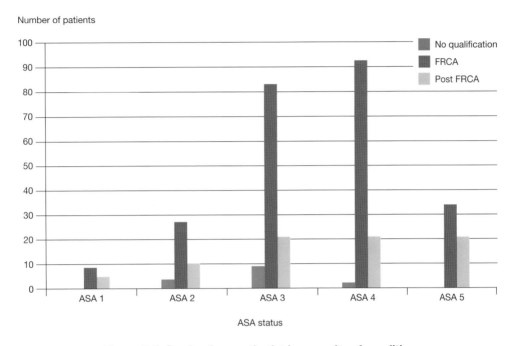

Figure 5.7. Grade of anaesthetist by severity of condition

For patients with worse health status (higher ASA score) it was more likely that more experienced anaesthetists were involved in the care. This represents good practice, however, ASA 3 and above should be cared for either directly or certainly under close supervision by senior anaesthetists[17] (Figure 5.7) Those without a higher diploma where not involved as the lead anaesthetist in the sickest of patients.

Single-handed anaesthetists

In this sample 110 cases were anaesthetised by single-handed anaesthetists. (Single-handed refers to the presence of only one medically qualified anaesthetist) The majority were senior anaesthetists which can be seen in Table 5.14.

Table 5.14 Grade of anaesthetist working alone

Grade of anaesthetist	n
Consultant	44
SpR with a certificate of completion of training	5
SpR without a certificate of completion of training	11
Staff grade and associate specialist (SAS)	14
Foundation year 2 or senior house officer	2
Other	1
Subtotal	**77**
Not answered	33
Grand Total	**110**

The ASA status of the patients anaesthetised by single-handed anaesthetists was distributed about ASA 3 (Table 5.15). Equally the NCEPOD classification of these cases was split evenly between Immediate/Urgent and Expedited/Elective (Table 5.16). Even for experienced anaesthetists ASA 3, 4, and 5 patients present a challenge and a medically qualified assistant would be of great value.

Table 5.15 Frequency of cases of an anaesthetist working alone by severity of the patients' condition

ASA status	n	%
Normal Healthy patient	2	1.8
Mild systemic disease	14	12.8
Severe systemic disease	52	47.7
Incapacitating systemic disease	30	27.5
Moribund	11	10.1
Subtotal	109	
Not answered	1	
Grand Total	110	

Table 5.16 Frequency of cases of an anaesthetist working alone by urgency of the procedure

Classification of operation	n	%
Immediate	15	13.8
Urgent	47	43.1
Expedited	20	18.3
Elective	27	24.8
Subtotal	109	
Not answered	1	
Grand Total	110	

The cases where single-handed anaesthetists cared for patients occurred mainly during the working day (8:00 -17:59).

Case study 10

An elderly patient presented to a district general emergency department with a dense left sided weakness and a Glasgow Coma Score of 7/15. Following intubation of the trachea and Intermittent Positive Pressure Ventilation a CT scan showed a large intracerebral cystic lesion causing mass effect. A cerebral abscess was suspected and the patient was transferred to the local neurosurgical centre. On arrival at the neurosurgical centre the patient underwent a stereotactic drainage of an intracerebral abscess at 01:00. The operating surgeon and anaesthetist were both senior specialist registrars. They had both, independently, sought advice from the on-call consultants. The patient developed septicaemia postoperatively and in the face of multiple comorbidities and a failure to respond to conventional therapies treatment was withdrawn.

The advisors believed that this was an example of an appropriate use of out of hours theatres and non consultant grade staff seeking advice.

Lead anaesthetist

The Royal College of Anaesthetists document *'Guidelines for the Provision of Anaesthetic Services'* states that:

"All medical services to patients, including anaesthetic services, provided in the National Health Service (NHS) are the responsibility of consultants …Trainee and non-consultant career grade (NCCG) or Staff and Associate Specialist (SAS) anaesthetists providing anaesthetic services must be supervised by a consultant."[13]

Case study 11

An elderly patient was admitted for an elective transurethral resection of prostate. He had suffered a previous myocardial infarction with subsequent coronary artery bypass graft surgery. He was hypertensive and had pleural effusions. The patient was graded ASA 3. An SAS anaesthetist did not seek advice. On review the patient had lateral T wave changes on a pre-operative ECG. Throughout the procedure the patient's systolic blood pressure was not above 90 mmHg. The patient was on warfarin which was stopped only three days pre-operatively.

The advisors were of the opinion that the anaesthetist involved should have sought the help and advice of a more senior clinician during the care of this patient.

Failing to record this on the anaesthetic record can be considered a fundamental failure by any hospital, as it will ensure that all key personnel involved in the care of a patient are named. The joint Royal College of Anaesthetists and the Association of Anaesthetists publication *'Good Practice'* refers to the levels of supervision in Part 1 of the College's CCT documents:

*"**Direct supervision:** Immediately available in the theatre or available in the theatre suite and without other responsibilities or*
*indirect supervision: Local – on the same geographical site and able to attend within 10 minutes; **Distant** – on a different geographical site or unable to attend within 10 minutes."*[11]

The lead anaesthetist was not a consultant in only 40 cases although grade of anaesthetist was not always recorded. If the lead anaesthetist was not a consultant, the advisors were asked if they thought that supervision was appropriate.

Table 5.17 Advisors' opinion of whether the supervision was appropriate when a consultant was not the lead anaesthetist

Appropriate supervision	n
Yes	10
No	6
Subtotal	**16**
Unable to answer	24
Grand Total	**40**

The advisors were only able to answer in 16 out of 40 cases.

Anaesthetic chart

The GMC impress on medical practitioners the need to keep"...*clear, accurate, legible and contemporaneous notes...*"[17]

Advisors were asked to grade the anaesthetic chart on the case notes by the following standards:
Good practice - All aspects of the documentation were well presented and easy to read
Satisfactory - Most aspects of the documentation were well presented and easy to read
Poor - Many aspects of the documentation were presented unclearly and difficult to read
Unacceptable - Unable to read a majority of the documentation

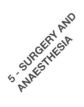
Table 5.18 Quality of the anaesthetic chart

Quality of the anaesthetic chart	n	%
Good	172	57.3
Satisfactory	116	38.7
Poor	5	1.7
Unacceptable	7	2.3
Subtotal	**300**	
Not answered	174	
Grand Total	**474**	

A total of 4.0% (12/300) of anaesthetic charts were considered poor or unacceptable (Table 5.18). This could not be assessed in 174/474 cases as the anaesthetic chart was not received by NCEPOD. NCEPOD has previously reported on the wide variability in the quality of medical notes as have the NHS Litigation Authority[18] and this study continues to demonstrate the importance of this theme. The King's Fund has also set a standard for health records in its Organisational Standards criteria, which states:

"There is an accurate health record which enables the patient to receive effective continuing care, enables the health care team to communicate effectively, allows another doctor or professional members of staff to assume care of the patient at any time, enables the patient to be identified without risk or error, facilitates the collection of data for research, education and audit and can be used in legal proceedings."[19]

If this standard of record keeping is not maintained and professional requirements are not being met, patients, and possibly staff, are put at risk. It cannot be emphasised too strongly that in medico-legal cases the outcome is often dependent on the anaesthetic record. An untidy, illegible, scantily completed chart may be taken as indirect evidence of poor care. Furthermore, the examination of medical records forms part of the GMC's fitness to practise procedures. The record must be such that if another doctor were required to take over the case, this record would allow systematic and ready access to all the information required.

Monitoring

The advisors considered that monitoring during the anaesthesia had been inadequate in 19 cases (Table 5.19).

Table 5.19 Adequate monitoring during anaesthesia – advisors' view

Adequate anaesthetic monitoring	n	%
Yes	295	93.9
No	19	6.1
Subtotal	**314**	
Insufficient data	160	
Grand Total	**474**	

For one case where the monitoring was deemed to be inadequate the missing monitoring was central venous pressure.

The same standards of monitoring apply when the anaesthetist is responsible for a local /regional anaesthetic or sedative technique for an operative procedure. The following monitoring devices are essential to the safe conduct of anaesthesia:
- pulse oximeter;
- non invasive blood pressure monitor;
- electrocardiograph;
- airway gases: oxygen, carbon dioxide and vapour;
- airway pressure.

If it is necessary to continue anaesthesia without a particular device, the anaesthetist must clearly record the reasons for this in the anaesthetic record[20].

Temperature maintenance

In 2008 the National Institute for Health and Clinical Excellence (NICE) stated that inadvertent peri-operative hypothermia is a common but preventable complication which is associated with poor outcomes. Prevention of inadvertent peri-operative hypothermia requires the use of simple measures to keep patients comfortably warm, alongside more active interventions such as forced air warming and fluid warming in the intra-operative phase[21]. It should be noted that the data for this study were collected prior to the issue of this guideline. However, methods were used to maintain patient's temperature in 89% (234/263) of cases in this study. Intravenous fluid warmers and warm air systems were the commonest mode of maintaining patient's peri-operative temperature.

Airway problems

Table 5.20 Airway problems – advisors' view

Airway problems	n	%
Yes	27	8.5
No	292	91.5
Subtotal	319	
Insufficient data	155	
Grand Total	474	

In the view of the advisors there were problems with the management of the airway in 27 cases (Table 5.20). The advisors were of the opinion that most were managed appropriately.

Appropriate postoperative analgesia

Table 5.21 Appropriate postoperative analgesia – advisors' view

Appropriate postoperative analgesia	n	%
Yes	253	95.5
No	12	4.5
Subtotal	265	
Insufficient data	209	
Grand Total	474	

Case study 12

An elderly patient with shortness of breath and stridor, unable to speak presented with swelling in the neck which had appeared over 24 hours. The patient was normally self caring and mobile. Apart from rheumatoid arthritis, no other history of note nor medication was recorded. The patient was unable to lie back and had to sit forward. Oxygen saturation was 94% on oxygen and 80% on air. Chest x-ray showed mediastinal shadowing and large heart. A provisional diagnosis of heart failure was made. The patient had been seen at 18:35 on arrival. At 20:38 the patient became distressed in resus and was unable to breath. Airway obstruction was suspected and they were moved to theatre. A senior anaesthetist was unable to intubate the patient at the first attempt due to blood in the airway. Cricothyroidotomy proved unsuccessful. A rigid bronchoscope provided an airway with subsequent intubation. The patient suffered a cardiac arrest and subsequently died. An autopsy showed a spontaneous haemorrhage into the soft tissues of the neck.

The advisors felt that this airway problem might have been recognised earlier. Stridor is a symptom that must not be underestimated. Early senior assessment is essential. Advanced airway management techniques may be needed and an ear, nose and throat surgical presence when managing the airway should be mandatory.

It was the advisors' view that the majority of patients (95.5%) received appropriate analgesia in the immediate postoperative period (Table 5.21).

Key findings

68.8% of patients had documented pre-operative assessment

91.5% (280/306) of cases had comorbidities that were managed adequately in the pre-operative period

95.8% of these sick patients were anaesthetised by an anaesthetist of the appropriate grade for their condition.

Frequently trainees and associate specialist anaesthetists did not record the consultant to whom they were responsible.

89% of patients had their temperature managed actively during the operative period.

Recommendations

Anaesthetic charts should routinely have a section that allows the recording of anaesthetic information (leaflets received, risks etc.) given to patients. (Clinical Directors)

Anaesthetic charts should record the named consultant and the grade of the anaesthetist anaesthetising the patient. (Clinical Directors and Consultants)

All trainees and staff and associate specialist grades should record the name and location of a supervising consultant and whether they have discussed the case with that consultant. (Clinical Directors and Consultants)

6 - General clinical issues

Investigations

Excludes paediatrics		
Clinical questionnaire	Total population	3059
	Population where radiological investigation performed	2379
Assessment form	Total population	2225
Organisational questionnaire		297

Following appropriate clinical assessment the management of the acutely ill patient relies on appropriate investigations being performed. Such investigations include radiology, biochemistry and physiological investigations. These should be timely and without delay. It is also important that resources and time are not spent on undertaking inappropriate tests. The advisors studied the data surrounding the investigations requested looking specifically at these issues.

Table 6.1 All essential investigations performed – advisors' opinion

All essential investigations performed	n	%
Yes	1899	91.3
No	182	8.7
Subtotal	2081	
Insufficient data	144	
Grand Total	2225	

Table 6.1 shows that the advisors found that most patients had appropriate investigations performed relevant to the nature and severity of their condition but in 8.7% (182/2081) did not.

Table 6.2 Outcome affected by omission of investigations – advisors' opinion

Outcome affected	n	%
Yes	83	4.4
No	1800	95.6
Subtotal	1883	
Insufficient data	342	
Grand Total	2225	

For 83/1883 patients the omission of investigations were thought by advisors to have affected the outcome (Table 6.2). The advisors made specific reference to many of the omitted investigations being related to organising radiological tests and this is covered in greater depth later in this section. Comparison to the 2007 report *'Emergency Admissions: A Journey in the Right Direction?'* shows a similar proportion of patients securing appropriate investigations.

Table 6.3 Delay in investigations being undertaken

Delay in investigations	n	%
Yes	107	5.2
No	1932	94.8
Subtotal	**2039**	
Unable to answer	126	
Not answered	60	
Grand Total	**2225**	

Table 6.3 shows that 107/2039 patients (5.2%) experienced a delay in the relevant investigations being performed and furthermore, 3.7% (75/2022) of patients experienced a delay in obtaining the results of such investigations (Table 6.4).

Table 6.4 Delay in obtaining investigations – advisors' opinion

Delay in obtaining investigations	n	%
Yes	75	3.7
No	1947	96.3
Subtotal	**2022**	
Insufficient data	203	
Grand Total	**2225**	

No patient should be put at risk by such delays. All relevant investigations should be organised at the time of admission and there should be no appreciable delay in getting results back. Good acute clinical care is based on the rapid assessment of patients. If broad physiological parameters, as defined by appropriate investigations, remain unknown owing to system failures then patients' lives are put at risk.

Radiology

Radiological investigations provide vital diagnostic information, can detail the extent of pathological findings and monitor response to therapy. In addition interventional radiological techniques have an increasing role to play in the management of many patients, replacing older surgical techniques. It was estimated in 2002 that approximately 30 million radiology investigations were carried out annually[22]. However it is known that there are significant year on year increases in demand, particularly in CT, MRI and interventional radiology. Patients rightly expect prompt and competent examination and treatment. This applies whether patients are seriously ill, have less life threatening undiagnosed conditions or simple fractures.

In this study radiological investigations were performed in 2379 patients. Only 605 patients had no radiological investigations and we could not tell from the data returned in 30 patients. In 45 cases the clinician completing the questionnaire did not indicate whether the patient had undergone radiological examinations or not.

The most common radiological investigations performed are listed in Table 6.5.

Table 6.5 Radiological exam requested

Radiological exam requested	n
Chest x-ray	1716
Abdominal x-ray/ultrasound	524
CT head	273
CT abdomen	189

Appropriateness of the radiological investigation

NCEPOD has previously commented on interventions being undertaken on patients not likely to benefit from the intervention or survive their illness.

Table 6.6 Radiological exam performed by expectation of survival

Expectation of survival	Radiology requested	n	%
Not expected to survive	Yes	1087	73.1
	No	384	25.8
	Unknown	17	1.1
	Subtotal	**1488**	
	Not answered	17	
Uncertain	Yes	962	86.7
	No	141	12.7
	Unknown	6	<1
	Subtotal	**1109**	
	Not answered	11	
Expected	Yes	306	78.7
	No	77	19.8
	Unknown	6	1.5
	Subtotal	**389**	
	Not answered	8	
Not answered	Yes	24	
	No	3	
	Subtotal	**27**	
	Unknown	1	
	Not answered	9	
Grand Total		**3059**	

Table 6.7 Radiology use by health status

Health status on admission	Radiology requested	n	%
Normal healthy patient	Yes	42	87.5
	No	5	10.4
	Unknown	1	2.1
	Subtotal	**48**	
	Not answered	1	
Mild systemic disease	Yes	203	87.1
	No	29	12.4
	Unknown	1	<1
	Subtotal	**233**	
	Not answered	3	
Severe systemic disease	Yes	600	83.1
	No	118	16.3
	Unknown	4	<1
	Subtotal	**722**	
	Not answered	14	
Incapacitating systemic disease	Yes	1046	79.9
	No	255	19.5
	Unknown	8	<1
	Subtotal	**1309**	
	Not answered	11	
A moribund patient	Yes	426	68.8
	No	184	29.7
	Unknown	9	1.5
	Subtotal	**619**	
	Not answered	10	
Not answered	Yes	62	
	No	14	
	Unknown	7	
	Subtotal	**83**	
	Not answered	6	
Grand Total		**3059**	

It appears from the data presented in the Tables 6.6 and 6.7 that many radiological investigations were being undertaken in moribund patients and patients not expected to survive their illness. This raises questions about appropriateness of these investigations with respect to both patient care and resource utilisation.

It was the opinion of the advisors that appropriate radiology investigations were undertaken in 1733 cases (96%) (Table 6.8).

Table 6.8 Appropriate investigations performed

Appropriate investigations	n	%
Yes	1733	96.0
No	73	4.0
Subtotal	1806	
Insufficient data	419	
Grand Total	2225	

Timing of radiological investigation
As most of the study population were emergency admissions the initial radiology investigations were often performed out of hours.

Table 6.9 Radiology performed out of hours

Performed out of hours	n	%
Yes	1241	53.8
No	982	42.6
Unknown	84	3.6
Subtotal	2307	
Not answered	72	
Grand Total	2379	

In this study 1241 out of 2307 investigations were performed out of hours (Table 6.9). This may have implications on staffing and availability of facilities if a comprehensive service is to be delivered on site[23].

Organisational data

Time to access appropriate investigations will be influenced by availability of services. Some diagnostic services may be available but without 24 hour cover.

Table 6.10 Conventional radiology

Conventional radiology	n	%
Not available	5	1.7
24 hours	260	89.9
<24 hours	24	8.3
Subtotal	289	
Not answered	8	
Grand Total	297	

Table 6.11 CT scanner

CT scanner	n	%
Not available	43	15.1
24 hours	198	69.7
<24 hours	43	15.1
Subtotal	284	
Not answered	13	
Grand Total	297	

Table 6.12 MRI scanner

MRI scanner	n	%
Not available	51	18.1
24 hours	81	28.8
<24 hours	149	53.0
Subtotal	281	
Not answered	16	
Grand Total	297	

Table 6.13 Angiography – non cardiac

Angiography - non cardiac	n	%
Not available	126	45.7
24 hours	76	27.5
<24 hours	74	26.8
Subtotal	276	
Not answered	21	
Grand Total	297	

Organisational data on the availability of conventional radiology, CT scanning, MRI scanning and non-cardiac angiography is shown in Tables 6.10 to 6.13. Five sites had no availability to perform conventional radiology (two of which were independent, one a small multiservice, one an acute specialist hospital and one not answered) and another 23 sites (six of which were independent) did not have 24 hour availability. The use of CT scanning has expanded greatly in recent years and advances in urgent/ emergency care is likely to see this continue (whole body imaging in trauma, thrombolysis in stroke for example). It is notable that 86 sites did not have access or had limited access to onsite CT scanning (Table 6.11). Inequality of access to interventional radiology services has been a recurring finding in NCEPOD reports[3,24] it is remarkable to find that so many hospitals still have no or limited access to angiography (Table 6.14).

Table 6.14 No or limited access to CT Scanning

Type of hospital	n
Acute specialist	10
Acute teaching	3
Large acute	4
Medium multiservice	2
Small acute	7
Small multiservice	9
Children's services	1
Independent	42
Multiple answers	3
Subtotal	81
Not answered	5
Grand Total	86

Reporting of first radiological investigation

The first documented report of a radiological investigation was the final report in 742 cases and a provisional report in 996 cases (Table 6.15).

Table 6.15 Type of report produced

Documentation of first report	n	%
Provisional report	996	57.3
Final report	742	42.7
Subtotal	1738	
Not answered	641	
Grand Total	2379	

Table 6.16 Type of report produced depending on whether the investigation was performed out of hours

Out of hours procedure	First documentation of report	n	%
Yes	Provisional	580	61.6
	Final report	362	38.4
	Subtotal	**942**	
	Not answered	299	
No	Provisional	382	52.3
	Final report	349	47.7
	Subtotal	**731**	
	Not answered	251	
Unknown	Provisional	20	
	Final report	23	
	Subtotal	**43**	
	Not answered	41	
Not answered	Provisional	14	
	Final report	8	
	Subtotal	**22**	
	Not answered	50	
Grand Total		**2379**	

Where investigations were performed out of hours (1241 cases) the report was provisional in 580 cases and final in 362 cases (Table 6.16). Provisional reports may be issued because staff reporting investigations are under consultant radiologist supervision (e.g. SpRs and sonographers) or because image manipulation is required before a final report can be issued (e.g. 3D reformats of complex pelvic fractures).

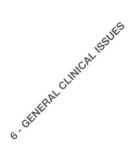

Table 6.17 Documentation of the report in the case notes

	Was the report documented in the case notes	n	%
Provisional report	Yes	853	86.6
	No	101	10.3
	Unknown	31	3.1
	Subtotal	**985**	
	Not answered	11	
Final report	Yes	446	60.8
	No	257	35.0
	Unknown	31	4.2
	Subtotal	**734**	
	Not answered	8	
Not answered	Yes	123	
	No	224	
	Unknown	57	
	Subtotal	**404**	
	Not answered	237	
Grand Total		**2379**	

It appears that provisional reports were more likely to be documented in the case notes than final reports; 35% of final and 10.3% of provisional reports were not recorded in the case notes (Table 6.17).

The difference between the documentation of preliminary and final reports in the notes may be expected. Preliminary reports are often handwritten and will be filed in the notes, but liable to loss as the patient moves around the hospital in the early phase of their care. The final report is typed and often viewed on the electronic patient record system rather than on paper copy and some departments no longer issue paper reports. The responsibility then is for ward based or medical records systems to file a report copy. We are currently at a transition point between paper based and IT based systems which is a potential source of information loss.

Where the report was documented in the notes this was written by a radiologist in 423 cases but by other clinicians in 952 cases (Table 6.18)

Table 6.18 Cases in which a radiologist documented the findings in the case notes

Designation of clinician writing the report	n	%
Radiologist	423	30.8
Other	952	69.2
Subtotal	1375	
Not answered	47	
Grand Total	1422	

It would appear that the standards laid down by the Royal College of Radiologists for communication of results are not being adhered to[25]. It is recognised that communication of the result of a radiology investigation is an important source of error[26] and harm[27] and it is recognised that better systems need to be put in place to overcome this important patient safety issue[28]. IT solutions already exist for these problems. Electronic order communication, voice recognition automated transcription, electronic priority labelling of reports and electronic logging report being read should eliminate these problems. This is one of a number of the drivers for their procurement but in the meantime robust systems should be established[25].

Appropriate patient management requires the input of senior and experienced clinicians. This applies equally to the requesting of investigations. Table 6.19 shows the seniority of clinician requesting the first radiology investigation. 47.6% of investigations were requested by F2/SHO or more junior doctors. These data do not allow discrimination between independent requests and those under the direction of more senior doctors.

Table 6.19 Grade of doctor requesting the investigation

Grade requesting exam	n	%
Consultant	307	16.1
SpR	477	24.9
SAS	100	5.2
F2 or SHO	911	47.6
F1 or HO	104	5.4
Nurse	3	<1
Other	10	<1
Subtotal	1912	
Not answered	467	
Grand Total	2379	

Radiological investigations usually have greatest value when new diagnostic findings which alter the management plan are identified. However negative investigations can also help by ruling out certain diagnoses.

Table 6.20 The effect of the outcome of the investigation on the patients' management

Management changed	n	%
Yes	564	27.1
No	1376	66.1
Unknown	143	6.9
Subtotal	2083	
Not answered	296	
Grand Total	2379	

In this study the radiological report changed management in 564 cases (27.1%) (Table 6.20).

Table 6.21 Timeliness of investigations – advisors' opinion

Timely investigations	n	%
Yes	1592	94.6
No	91	5.4
Subtotal	1683	
Insufficient data	542	
Grand Total	2225	

It was judged that in 91 cases (5.4%) investigations were not performed in a timely manner (Table 6.21).

It has previously been shown by the Audit Commission that approximately 20% of radiology investigations did not help patient care[22] and whilst the question asked within this study may not exactly mirror that asked by the Audit Commission it appears that many investigations do not change the management of patient care in this group of patients who died. Better use of the radiology resource may be realised by better use of referral guidelines[29], checking and discussion of requests and use of multidisciplinary meetings and teams.

It was stated that in seven cases more rapid access to the final report or review with a clinician would have altered outcome (Table 6.22).

Table 6.22 Effect on outcome assessed by speed of review

Rapid review would have altered outcome	n	%
Yes	7	<1
No	1941	90.0
Unknown	63	2.9
Not applicable	146	6.8
Subtotal	2157	
Not answered	222	
Grand Total	2379	

Table 6.23 Discrepancies between the provisional and the final report

Final report differed from the initial report	n	%
Yes	40	2.2
No	1199	65.5
Unknown	592	32.3
Subtotal	1831	
Not answered	548	
Grand Total	2379	

The final report differed from the provisional report in 40 cases (Table 6.23). This appears to be a small number (2.2%) but it was unknown or unanswered in 1140 cases. The advisors commented that the frequency of discrepancies between provisional and final reports was likely to be much higher and that there was no robust mechanism to capture the differences between provisional and final reports. It is recommended that where a report has been altered the final report clearly documents this.

Table 6.24 Formal investigation discussed with the team caring for the patient

Investigation formally discussed	n	%
Yes	1018	50.0
No	613	30.1
Unknown	407	20.0
Subtotal	2038	
Not answered	341	
Grand Total	2379	

The investigation was formally discussed at a meeting or had additional clinical involvement in 1018 cases (Table 6.24). The advisors commented that good clinical liaison allowed more accurate radiological advice by ensuring good clinical information and context. Again there was a high number of unknown/unanswered cases, further strengthening the impression that documentation of radiology involvement is less than ideal.

Key findings

182 patients did not have all essential investigations performed.

5% of patients had a delay in their investigations being performed.

96% of patients who underwent a radiological investigation had all appropriate radiological investigations performed.

1241/2338 (53.1%) of initial radiological investigations were performed out of hours.

Access to CT scanning and MRI scanning is a substantial problem with many sites having no or limited (<24hours) on site provision.

Only 150/297 hospitals have on site angiography (non-cardiac) and of these only 76 have 24 hour access.

Recommendations

All admissions to hospital should have appropriate investigations and these should be performed without unnecessary delay. (Consultants)

Hospitals which admit patients as an emergency must have access to plain radiology and CT scanning 24 hours per day, with immediate reporting (This recommendation was previously reported in *'Emergency Admissions: A Journey in the Right Direction?'* in 2007). (Medical Directors)

There should be robust mechanisms to ensure communication of critical, urgent or unexpected radiological findings in line with guidance issued by the Royal College of Radiologists. (Clinical Directors)

Diagnostic and interventional radiology services should be adequately resourced to support the 24 hour needs of their clinicians and patients. (Clinical Directors)

Any difference between the provisional and final radiology report should be clearly documented in the final report. (Consultants)

Venous thromboembolism

Excludes paediatrics		Denominator
Clinical questionnaire	Total population	3059
	Admitted under a surgeon	1354
	Admitted under a physician	1442
	Unable to determine admitting specialty	263

Prophylaxis against venous thromboembolus (VTE) remains an area where practice is less than ideal. Although the audit period preceded publication of the recent NICE Guideline[30] for surgical patients on this topic circulation of the draft guidance coincided with the start of data collection. Thus clinicians should have been alerted to a drive to increase compliance with this important aspect of therapy.

The fact that the Guideline is primarily directed at surgical patients highlights the urgent need for a similar document covering the management of acute medical patients. Perhaps this is the reason why surgeons, in the main, were more aggressive in prescribing prophylaxis with 52.2% (670/1283) of the patients included in this study receiving some form of intervention (where this was known) compared to only 34% (464/1365) of acute medical admissions. The data are summarised in Table 6.25. Nevertheless we cannot ignore the fact that only 1225/2868 (42.7%) from the whole study definitely received prophylaxis.

Table 6.25 Venous thromboembolism precautions taken by specialty

	Total population		Admitted by a surgeon		Admitted by a physician		Unknown
VTE precautions taken	n	%	n	%	n	%	n
Yes	1225	42.7	670	52.2	464	34.0	91
No	1333	46.5	481	37.5	753	55.2	99
Unknown	310	10.8	132	10.3	148	10.8	30
Subtotal	**2868**		**1283**		**1365**		**220**
Not answered	191		71		77		43
Grand Total	**3059**		**1354**		**1442**		**263**

Amongst surgical specialties adherence to some form of prophylaxis protocol was greatest amongst trauma and orthopaedic patients, an area where there has been considerable reluctance to institute such regimens in the past. This reluctance reflected concerns about haematoma formation and an increased risk of infection in operations in which a prosthesis had been implanted. The data for surgical patients is shown in Table 6.26.

Table 6.26 Venous thromboembolism precautions taken by surgical specialty

Admitting specialty	VTE precautions taken	n	%
General surgery	Yes	374	51.6
	No	280	38.6
	Unknown	71	9.8
	Subtotal	**725**	
	Not answered	36	
Trauma and orthopaedics	Yes	158	73.1
	No	35	16.2
	Unknown	23	10.6
	Subtotal	**216**	
	Not answered	11	8.8
Grand Total		**988**	

However, further inspection of the data revealed that low molecular weight heparin (LMWH) was prescribed less often for trauma and orthopaedic patients (65.8% of those receiving prophylaxis 104/158) compared to general surgical patients (87.3%; 309/354) and thus this concern may still persist. This was of interest given that the NICE Guideline referred to above recommends a combination of mechanical prophylaxis (graduated elasticated compression stockings, calf stimulators or foot pumps) in combination with LMWH or fondaparinux (a similar anticoagulant) in patients with hip fractures.

The surgical data also revealed that a substantial proportion of general surgical patients in whom prophylaxis was provided were given both LMWH and graduated elasticated compression stockings since the latter were prescribed for 58% of the prophylaxis group. In orthopaedic and trauma patients there was greater reliance on a single method of prevention (Table 6.27).

The scope of this report did not allow us to determine the nature of any formal policy that was in place for DVT prophylaxis in the contributing institutions. Although LMWH was widely prescribed the recent NICE Guideline places more emphasis on the use of mechanical methods (graduated elasticated compression stockings ±calf stimulators or foot pumps) in surgical patients except for those at a higher risk of VTE (malignancy, cardiac or respiratory failure, acute medical illness, immobility, obesity etc) and those undergoing orthopaedic procedures. In these groups mechanical prevention should be supplemented by LMWH.

Whilst it may appear that there was a higher use of LMWH than anticipated by the new Guideline the majority of patients were admitted as emergencies with an acute illness thus placing them in a high-risk group for VTE. This reflects the need for more aggressive preventative measures.

For medical patients only 34% (464/1365) of patients received any form of prophylaxis with LMWH prescribed in 370/464 of these. This appears unacceptably low given the high prevalence of major risk factors for VTE (active cardiac or respiratory failure, acute medical illness, age over 60 years, recent myocardial infarction or stroke, sepsis).

Table 6.27 Method of venous thromboembolism precaution used by surgical specialty

Specialty admitted under	Method of precaution	n
General surgery	Heparin	309
	Graduated elasticated compression stockings	218
	Heparin and Graduated elasticated compression stockings	171
	Calf compressions	29
	Other	9
Trauma and orthopaedics	Heparin	104
	Graduated elasticated compression stockings	71
	Heparin and Graduated elasticated compression stockings	43
	Calf compressions	19
	Other	28

*Answers may be multiple

Key findings

Patients admitted under a surgeon appeared to be more likely to receive venous thromboembolism prophylaxis. Nevertheless, only 55% of patients admitted under a surgeon and 38% of patients admitted under a physician did so.

The use of venous thromboembolism prophylaxis in medical patients included in this study was unacceptably low.

National guidelines for prophylaxis in medical patients are being developed and urgently required.

7 - Paediatric care

	Denominator
Clinical questionnaire	94
Assessment form	77
Anaesthetic questionnaire	3

Babies, children and young people make up an estimated 20% of the population of the UK[31]. Mortality outside the neonatal period is around 2.5/10,000[32], with post neonatal mortality being one of the highest in Europe[33]. The anticipated number of deaths in the 4 week to 16 year range in this study was small in comparison with adults. However, it should be noted that the rate of deaths was higher in this group than in the group of patients aged 16-25 years. This was thought to be due to deaths in childhood which occurred secondary to the effects of prematurity, congenital malformation and severe infection. NCEPOD[34] along with other review teams[32,35] have pointed to the fact that remediable factors are often present in childhood deaths. There are factors that are common to all age groups, and others which are relevant to babies and children, and which deserve particular discussion and comment.

Demographics

Within this section the term paediatric is used to indicate the full age range i.e. babies (infants < 1 year), children and young people (up to age 16). This study excluded neonates (0-28 days).

There were a total of 94 clinical questionnaires returned in the under 16 age range (38 female and 56 in male), with 45 under the age of two years, including 19 in infancy. Case notes were returned for 77 patients. This age distribution is in keeping with a recent pilot study of childhood deaths 0-18 in 5 UK regions in 2006[34], in which about a quarter of deaths were in babies aged less than one year.

Cause of death

Most admissions were classified as medical (79) with only 10/94 being classed as surgical (five patients had surgery) and in five patients the specialty was not recorded. This is in keeping with other work on deaths in the paediatric population. Peri-operative death in children is the subject of a forthcoming study by NCEPOD and will therefore not be reviewed here in detail.

The profile of diagnoses at death was diverse. It is important to note that:

1. Many children had comorbidity on admission, 55 having moderate or severe incapacitating systemic disease (as defined by the ASA scores 3 and 4).

2. Respiratory disease including pneumonia and acute severe asthma were relatively common with a total of 13 deaths with a clear precipitating respiratory illness. This is unsurprising as overall respiratory disease causes 15% of hospital admissions and an estimated 8% of deaths in childhood[36]. Although asthma deaths in childhood have remained static since the early 1990s, they still occur[37-39] and asthma is more prevalent in the UK than other European countries.

3. Severe infections were directly associated with 12 deaths, including 6 cases of encephalitis and meningitis.

Case study 13

A very young child with an acute exacerbation of severe asthma was admitted after discussions between parents and the paediatric team. The family had 'open access' to the unit. On admission oxygen saturation was recorded as 72% in air and nursing staff administered further nebulisers and oxygen with improvement in saturations. A junior paediatrician was delayed in seeing the child and when placing an intravenous cannula to administer aminophlylline the child struggled and had a respiratory and then cardiac arrest from which they could not be resuscitated.

The advisors commented that there was likely to have been a lack of recognition of severity of illness in a child with severe chronic asthma, and that cannulation probably precipitated the respiratory arrest. No further information was available with regard to their chronic anaemia.

Routine immunisation against invasive pneumococcal disease was introduced in the UK in February 2006. Prior to this approximately 5000 cases occurred in England and Wales each year, with about 10% being in children under two years and about one third of these presenting as cases of meningitis[40]. It was estimated that about 10% of those under two years who contracted the disease died from it, and many more were left with serious disability. Our study looked at the whole of 2006, when it was likely that many babies and young children had not yet benefited from the vaccine. An additional important effect of immunisation is likely to be a reduction in resistant streptococcus pneumoniae infections, which has already been noted in North America where vaccine was available from 2002[41]. Immunisation for other very serious bacterial infections in childhood, namely haemophilus influenzae and meningitis C, was in place prior to 2006[42].

Case study 14

A very young child was admitted by direct GP referral after a 24 hour illness. The patient was noted to have a reduced conscious level (Glasgow Coma Score 3/15), poor peripheral perfusion (capillary refill 5 seconds) and a low blood sugar. A diagnosis of meningo-encephalitis was made, but despite prompt resuscitation, which included intubation, ventilation and referral to paediatric intensive care unit they developed seizures, signs of increasing intracranial pressure and brain stem death only eight hours after admission. A sample of cerebrospinal fluid taken after brain stem death had been declared, revealed streptococcus pneumoniae.

Advisors commented on the exemplary standard of care and documentation. Had a vaccine been available at this time the death should have been preventable. However streptococcus pneumoniae often has a poor prognosis, particularly when presenting late.

Overall quality of care

In the 77 cases where advisor assessment was possible, the overall quality of care was judged to be good in 55 (Figure 7.1). However there were 11 cases where there was believed to be room for improvement in clinical care, four cases where there could be improvements in organisational aspects of care, three cases where there could be improvements in both clinical and organisation aspects of care. In three cases care was felt to be less than satisfactory. In one case, there was insufficient data to assess the overall quality of care the patient had received.

Pathway of admission

About a third of paediatric patients (34/94) were admitted via the Emergency Department (ED). This is a smaller number than is reflected in the complete data set (i.e. that including adult deaths), in which about two thirds were admitted via the ED. A minority were admitted via GP referral (3), some were directly transferred from other units (15), and some self referred to wards and units (16). Parents and carers may perceive that severe illness in children is best dealt with in a hospital setting. There is

also evidence to suggest that since the change to the GP contract in 2001, there has been an increase in children attending EDs[43,44]. It is therefore clearly important that ED staff have and maintain appropriate competencies to deal with sick children[45].

The initial place of admission was an intensive care unit in about a third of paediatric patients in this study population (level 3 intensive care in 29 children, with 8 children admitted direct to level 2 intensive care). This was a relatively large proportion compared with adult medical patients. Whilst the majority of paediatric admissions to intensive care is appropriate for sick children, most UK hospitals care for very small numbers each year[46]. Many children are initially admitted to adult/general intensive care units (AICUs) are then transferred to regional paediatric intensive care units (PICUs), which in England, Wales and Scotland care for about 14,000 children under 16 per year with a mortality of about 5%[47]. Others will inevitably die in a District or University hospital setting before transfer can be arranged. This has important planning and resource implications for care of the critically ill child[48].

Number of patients

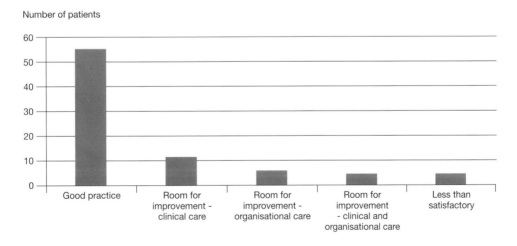

Figure 7.1 Overall quality of care of the paediatric group

Transfers

A third of paediatric cases in this study (31/92) were transferred at some point to another hospital (not answered in two cases). In the majority this was in order to receive specialist care including intensive care. All transfers were judged appropriate. However in 3/31 it was felt by the clinicians completing the questionnaire that transfer was delayed, but this did not appear to be to the detriment of overall care.

Team working, including time and degree of early senior input

In total 55/87 cases had their initial assessment performed by a SpR (31) or Consultant (24), (not answered = 7) and in 66 cases the diagnosis was made by a consultant. In 71 cases we found that the time from arrival to first assessment was < 1 hour.

Although review by a consultant was generally at an early stage, with 46 babies and children being seen by a consultant within two hours of admission, a small number (9/77) were not seen by a consultant within the first 12 hours. In three cases consultant review occurred > 24 hours after admission, and in two at 36-48 hours. In 17 cases no time to consultant review was given. Children who present very severely ill are relatively uncommon. They may have associated complex comorbidity which is likely to require input from experienced clinicians, who in turn may need to seek advice and assistance from other specialist colleagues.

Advisors believed that there was evidence of delays in consultant review in 4/63 paediatric cases (insufficient data to assess in 14 cases).

Furthermore, from the sample it could be seen that in 4/70 cases (insufficient data in 7 cases) there was a lack of a clear management plan and one of these also had a delayed consultant review.

Case study 15

A child who had received a heart transplant at the age of two presented to their local hospital febrile with a cough, increasing shortness of breath and a recent seizure which precipitated the admission. The patient's immunosuppressive medication had been reduced approximately one month previously due to high plasma drug levels. On examination the patient had chest signs, an enlarged liver and a base deficit of -20 on a first blood gas. A working diagnosis of sepsis was made and the patient was commenced on intravenous antibiotics, and referred to be seen by a local adult cardiologist, who believed that cardiac function was good. Sixteen hours after admission the patient had a further seizure and had a cardiac arrest from which they could not be resuscitated. An autopsy revealed gross evidence of previous cardiac ischaemia and acute rejection.

The advisors commented on the complexity of this patient's problems. There was no documentation of discussions with the tertiary centre during the admission. If this conversation had taken place, colleagues may have alerted clinicians to the possibility of organ rejection. A base deficit of -20 is always a cause for concern. Children and young people often compensate clinically until a relatively late stage of deterioration.

In 9/71 cases it was felt that there were omissions in the initial management plan, and in three of these the plan was also unclear (insufficient data to assess in 6 cases).

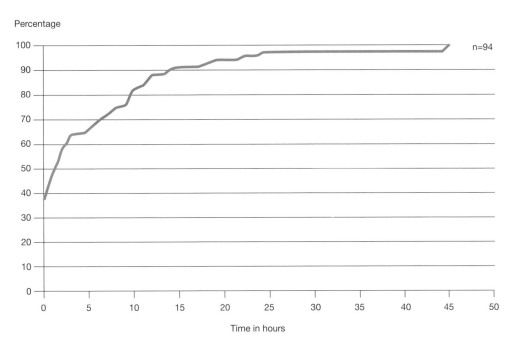

Percentage

n=94

Time in hours

Figure 7.2 Time in hours to consultant assessment

Ideally the timing of all assessments as well as the name and grade of assessor should be clearly recorded in the patient record, even if the severity of illness necessitates that attendants write this in retrospect. In 24/77 cases where a full set of records was provided it was not possible to ascertain the time of consultant assessments. Therefore data were taken from the medical/surgical questionnaire and presented in Figure 7.2 outlining the time to consultant review.

Just under half of the children in this study died in intensive care (32/76), (not answered in 1 case). Four children died in the operating theatre or recovery room of whom one had not undergone surgery. This was because the child had been transferred to this setting for resuscitation and stabilisation; a common practice in smaller hospitals without dedicated paediatric emergency departments or paediatric intensive care. Whilst such facilities can provide a perfectly adequate environment, staff, equipment and a full team approach is still required.

Case study 16

A very young child with multiple problems including severe developmental delay, chronic lung disease, ventriculo-peritoneal shunt and Hirschsprungs disease had been admitted to their local hospital within the previous three days with a diarrhoeal illness. The local hospital did not have a paediatric intensive care unit or a rota for specialist paediatric anaesthesia. They were re-admitted late in the evening with a high fever and oxygen saturations of 80%. The child was treated on the ward with oxygen therapy, intravenous fluids and antibiotic. At 08:50 the next day they had deteriorated and were transferred to theatre for intubation by a consultant anaesthetist. After intubation the patient proved difficult to ventilate with high inflation pressures, but oxygenation improved. However, while the tube was being changed the child arrested and could not be resuscitated. At no point was the patient attended by a consultant paediatrician.

Advisors' comments were that this child was sicker than appreciated by the middle grade paediatricians who cared for them, and that the child should have received airway intervention earlier. The anaesthetist should have had additional senior paediatric medical assistance in theatre.

Recognition of severity of illness

Only 11 children and young people were said to have no comorbidity or only mild systemic disease on admission, with the majority (76) suffering severe systemic disease or being moribund on admission.

As previously stated, in the main paediatric cases were seen early by a consultant, who often made the diagnosis. In 11/86 cases the first assessment was performed by ED staff, and in one by orthopaedics, (not answered in 8 cases). In four cases the diagnosis was made by an SHO or F2 doctor. It is particularly important that all grades and specialities are trained in the recognition of severe illness in children as well as adults, and involve senior personnel at an early stage in management[49]. The introduction of Paediatric Early Warning Scoring[50] into routine practice and from admission should be encouraged.

Height and weight data

Weight was recorded in a majority of cases, but was absent from notes in 23 children. However height or length was recorded in only 15 cases. Since drug and fluid doses are generally closely based on weight, we assume that this essential omission posed difficulties for attendants. It is appreciated that weighing very sick babies and children may be impossible. However in these circumstances it is accepted practice to make estimates[51,52]. In such cases it would be reasonable to expect that such an estimated weight to be clearly recorded.

End of life care

Forty five patients were not expected to survive on admission with 21 being classed as terminal and 24 non terminal.

Four patients had involvement of palliative care teams, and these cases were on the whole well managed. Twenty eight children and young people had a do not attempt resuscitation order in place and three an advance directive - six had both.

Discussions about withdrawal of treatment were in the majority of cases conducted with the family (66/77), (not answered in 17 cases). In 12/81 these were also with the child or young person, (not answered in 13 cases). However in 11/82 cases it would appear that discussions did not occur at all (not answered in 12 cases). This may have been appropriate (for example when cardiac arrest was unanticipated, resuscitation attempts unsuccessful, and parents were not present). Nevertheless, this should be rare, and parents need be included in discussions as a matter of routine practice. Many will also wish to be present during resuscitation. A review of children's palliative care services in 2007[53] pointed to the need for clear care pathways to be developed along the lines of those provided by the Association for Children's Palliative Care.

On admission 76 patients were suffering from either incapacitating systemic disease or deemed moribund (ASA 5). Ten of the 48 patients with incapacitating systemic disease and 17 of the 28 patients who were moribund were admitted to intensive care. Whilst it was felt by advisors that the majority of these admissions were appropriate, consideration should always be given to the risks and benefits of care, particularly if the patient is in the last stages of a terminal illness.

Morbidity and mortality meetings

It was notable that so few cases appeared to have been discussed at Morbidity and Mortality meetings, with advisors finding that in only 11/77 cases there was evidence of a meeting having taken place. There is now a mandatory system in England, Wales and Northern Ireland (from April 2008) whereby all "unexpected" deaths are reviewed by area child death review panels[54] under the auspices of Local Safeguarding Children Boards. This may mean that it is more likely in future that departments will have a system in place to peer review deaths. The most recent review of Safeguarding

in England has reinforced the need for all health care professionals to be aware of child protection issues, which may present as unexplained or unexpected death or serious injury[55]. NCEPOD recommended in 1999[36] that all peri-operative deaths in children should be the subject of multidisciplinary review. We are unsure how many departments comply with this.

Case study 17

A young child with complex needs including microcephaly, asthma, renal impairment and a previous paediatric intensive care unit (PICU) admission was re-admitted with pneumonia. During a previous stay on the PICU six months previously the child's parents had agreed that it would not be in the child's interests to undergo full resuscitation if they should arrest. The patient deteriorated ten hours after admission in the early hours of the morning and the parents then requested that the child undergo full treatment including PICU referral, which was accepted. The child arrested and died soon after intubation by the local team, despite prolonged efforts to resuscitate. The admitting consultant commented that it had been difficult to discuss a care plan with the child's parents between acute admissions as "the patient was not improving and getting towards the end of their life". The consultant felt that the parents were not ready for discussions which might have prepared them for the future.

The advisors stated that it was unfortunate that no plan was in place. The fact that latterly there was lack of recognition of the need for senior input into the decision making with this child was a particular issue.

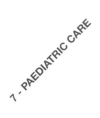
Key findings

Initial diagnosis was more often made by a consultant as compared with adult patients. NCEPOD recognises that recognition of serious illness in children is sometimes relatively difficult and requires the input of senior clinicians at the onset.

District hospitals may have particular problems delivering a high standard of care when dealing with very sick children and it is recognised that a well co-ordinated team approach is required.

A minority of paediatric deaths were in a surgical context. A forthcoming NCEPOD study will look at the care of such patients.

8 - End of life care

Excludes paediatrics		Denominator
Clinical questionnaire	Total population	3059
	Admitted under a surgeon	1354
	Admitted under a physician	1442
	Unable to determine admitting specialty	263
Assessment form	Total population	2225
Assessment form by clinical questionnaire		2090

The majority of people who die in the UK do so in acute hospitals usually following a chronic illness and are over the age of 75 years[56]. This is in marked contrast to the turn of the twentieth century when most people died in their own home following acute illness and were of a younger age group[57]. Over the last 100 years attitudes of both the general population and health care professionals has changed towards death and the care of the dying. While in the past death was very much considered "part of life", modern society has seemed less willing to discuss the issues surrounding death and dying. This has now been recognised and there has been increasing recognition especially over the last decade that end of life care needs to improve[58].

End of life care services are intended to ensure that patients have the best quality of life until they die. This care may be provided by a wide range of health care and social care providers, family members, friends and the voluntary sector. Furthermore specialist palliative care services provide end of life care in the hospital setting and in the community.

Most people would prefer to die in their own home even though less than 20% do, with a similar proportion of patients dying in care homes and very few patients dying in hospices[56]. While it may be appropriate for some patients to be admitted to acute hospitals to die, for many this is inappropriate. As a consequence in July 2008, following two years of consultation, the Department of Health (DH) published the 'End of Life Care Strategy' emphasising the need to improve end of life care services in the community, enhancing health and social care workers knowledge and skills and developing specialist palliative care services[59] and subsequently the National Audit Office has published 'End of Life Care'[60].

Department of Health's End of Life Care Strategy

Key areas to be addressed:

- Raising the profile of end of life care and changing attitudes to death and dying in society.
- Strategic commissioning to provide an integrated approach to the planning and delivery of end of life care services across health and social care, led by PCTs and local authorities.
- Identifying people approaching the end of life to allow a discussion about the person's preferences for the place and type of care needed.
- Care planning to assess the needs and wishes of the person and to agree the subsequent care plan with the person and their carer. The care plan should be available to all who have a legitimate reason to see it (for example, out of hours and emergency services).
- Coordination of care to ensure that each person approaching the end of life receives coordinated care, perhaps with a central coordinating facility providing a single point of access for people.
- Rapid access to care with medical and personal care and support for people 24 hours a day, seven days a week. The provision of these services should prevent emergency admissions to hospitals and enable more people approaching the end of their life to live and die in the place of their choice.
- Delivery of high quality services in all locations in the community, care homes, hospices, hospitals and ambulance services.
- Last days of life and care after death. The Liverpool Care Pathway or equivalent approach will be used to empower generalist clinicians to care for the dying and manage pain and other symptoms in the last days and hours of life, and to coordinate care after death.

- Involving and supporting carers in the provision of care. Carers may need practical and emotional support both during the person's life and in bereavement. Carers have the right to have their own needs assessed and reviewed.
- Education and training and continuing professional development to embed end of life care in training curricula, induction and continuing professional development for all registered and unregistered health and social care staff whether working full time on such care or not.
- Measurement and research of structure, process and outcomes of care to monitor care given and to develop further end of life care services. The Department of Health also wishes to enhance research into end of life care especially for those with conditions other than cancer.
- Funding. It is difficult to calculate the cost of end of life care across health and social care because of difficulties in defining the boundaries of such care and of identifying the cost to carers. The Department of Health has provided extra funding of £286 million for 2009-10 and 2010-11 but believes that many improvements can be made by better use of existing resources, for example by reductions in hospital admissions and length of stay.

As summarised in: End of Life Care. National Audit Office, Stationary Office, London, November 2008

National Audit Office: End of Life Care

Summary of the key recommendations:

- The wishes of people approaching the end of their life are not always conveyed to those who need to know. This information should be regularly updated and shared with all providers across the health, social care, independent and voluntary sectors.
- There are significant gaps in the education and training curricula for health and social care professionals. The Department of Health should work with the relevant professional bodies to ensure that all trainee doctors, nurses, allied health professionals, and registered social care staff receive an appropriate level of training in the delivery of end of life care. The General Medical Council's Education Committee in its review of Tomorrow's Doctors should address how to improve skills in identification, delivery, and awareness of end of life care. The review by the Nursing and Midwifery Council of pre-registration nursing education should address similar issues.
- Few care home staff have sufficient training in providing end of life care. The Department of Heath should strengthen the existing standards against which care homes are assessed to include a requirement to demonstrate that staff have received such training, including: communication skills; how to avoid unplanned emergency admissions; the provision of adequate pain management; and treating all residents with dignity and respect.
- The Gold Standards Framework, Liverpool Care Pathway and Preferred Priorities for Care provide a framework for improving the delivery of end of life care, including identifying the point at which it should begin. Little is known, however, about the direct patient benefits associated with their use. The Department of Health should commission clinical evaluations to determine whether their use results directly in better quality care for patients.

- Commissioning end of life care services is complex and there is a limited understanding of the national picture of demand and supply of end of life care services. The Department of Health should provide more information and, as appropriate, guidance to assist PCTs to meet end of life care needs and allocate resources more efficiently and effectively by building on the evidence from our work.
- Advance care plans seek to make clear a person's wishes in anticipation of a gradual deterioration in their condition, which may result in a loss of capacity to make decisions or to communicate their wishes to others. PCTs should encourage providers to develop care plans, including advance care plans, for those who wish to have one, and review and update them as necessary.
- A lack of coordination between services or a single point of contact can lead to frustration for patients and carers. PCTs should commission effective coordination of end of life care services through a single point of contact for patients and carers.
- PCTs generally contract with independent hospices on an annual basis leading to uncertainty in planning and sometimes financial pressures. PCTs should work with independent hospices to develop three year contracts, based on commissioned services and levels of activity, to enable hospices to better plan the use of resources.
- Hospitals will continue to have an important role to play in end of life care but these services do not always meet the needs of patients and carers. PCTs should use the World Class Commissioning Framework to commission end of life care services from hospitals to meet the needs of patients and carers.

Taken from: End of Life Care. National Audit Office, Stationary Office, London, November 2008

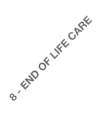

The sample of data collected in this current NCEPOD study was taken before the DH's *'End of Life Care Strategy'* was published and thus the findings will act as a valuable baseline of information of the state of end of life care in the UK. Data were collected on various aspects of end of life care from the clinical questionnaires although the majority of information collected came from the peer review of individual cases and the subsequent commentary of the advisors. It should be remembered that only patients who died within four days of admission were included and thus they may not represent all patients who were admitted with palliative intent. Furthermore some patients' management changed from curative to palliation following admission.

Expectation of survival

Before any form of end of life care can be commenced an assessment of the patient's life expectancy needs to be undertaken. The sample of patients included in this study all died within four days of admission although not all were expected to do so. The clinicians completing the clinical questionnaire were asked, following the initial assessment of the patient, the expected outcome of the patient (Table 8.1). For half of patients admitted 1505/3022 (49.8%) the clinicians who answered this question considered that the patients were not expected to survive; in 37 cases the question was not answered. Of these the clinicians further categorised them into two groups:

- those admitted and not expected to survive for terminal care which mainly included patients with cancer;
- those admitted, not expected to survive but not terminal care, the majority of these patients had end stage non cancer disease for example pulmonary, neurological, cardiac diseases and patients with inoperable surgical pathology.

For the 745/3022 (24.7%) patients admitted for terminal care, at a minimum one would expect some form of end of life care to be commenced and consideration given for a do not attempt resuscitation (DNAR) order.

Table 8.1 Expectation of survival on admission

Expectation of survival	n	%
Not expected (terminal care)	745	24.7
Not expected (not terminal care)	760	25.1
Uncertain	1120	37.1
Expected	397	13.1
Subtotal	**3022**	
Not answered	37	
Grand Total	**3059**	

The clinicians were also asked to describe the health care status of the patient on admission (Figure 8.1).

The majority of those patients with incapacitating disease or in a moribund state were considered not expected to survive. There was a slightly greater proportion (88%; 637/723) of these categories in the terminal care group compared to the not terminal care group (81%; 596/740). With such a large number of patients who had a poor prognosis the importance of discussion of treatment limitations with the patient and or relatives would be considered of upmost importance.

Necessity of admission and admission pathway

It has been suggested that as many has 40% of patients who are nearing the end of their lives are admitted inappropriately to acute hospitals to die[62]. Indeed in a previous NCEPOD report investigating patients who were admitted as an emergency to hospital, 5.9% of patients who died were considered to be unnecessary

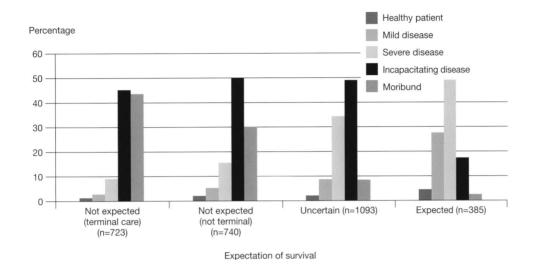

Figure 8.1 Health care status of patients by expectation of survival

admissions[3]. This figure underestimates the number of inappropriate admissions because only deaths within seven days of admission were included and patients admitted for palliative care were excluded. However, a common theme amongst these unnecessary admissions was that of elderly patients admitted for social reasons or patients with untreatable terminal conditions which should have been adequately managed in the community.

In this current study the clinicians completing the clinical questionnaire were asked if the admission was necessary. Of those that answered 128/2981 (4.2%) considered that the patients' admission was not necessary. In most cases (2845/2981) it was stated that the admission was necessary, and it was not answered in 86 cases. Table 8.2 shows the expectation of survival of those patients in whom the admission was unnecessary. Although the numbers are small one can see that most of these patients were for terminal care.

Table 8.2 Expectation of survival where admission was unnecessary

Expectation to survive	n	%
Not expected (terminal)	80	63.0
Not expected (not terminal)	32	25.2
Uncertain	11	8.7
Expected	4	3.1
Subtotal	**127**	
Not answered	1	
Grand Total	**128**	

Where it could be determined from the case notes the opinion of the advisors was also obtained as to the necessity of the admission. In 123/2090 (5.9%) of patients reviewed the admission was considered unnecessary (in 470 cases advisors didn't give details as to the overall assessment – 123/1620 7.6%). Again it should be borne in mind that this represents a subset of the total of possible unnecessary admissions because the patients in this study died within 4 days of admission.

As in *Emergency Admissions: A journey in the right direction?* NCEPOD 2007[3] reasons given by advisors for considering that admissions were inappropriate included:

- a deficiency of social and medical support in the home or nursing home;
- poor communication between health care and social providers e.g. in hours and out of hours GP services;
- poor systems for communicating treatment limitation intention e.g. advance directive and do not attempt resuscitation status;
- poor coordination of services of health care providers;
- lack of assessment and planning of end of life health care needs;
- inadequate access to community palliative care services.

The following case studies provide examples of some of these issues.

Case study 18

An elderly patient with advanced dementia and Parkinson's disease was sent to the emergency department from a nursing home on a Friday evening. The patient was unconscious, hypotensive, hypothermic and an ECG showed acute myocardial ischaemia. The patient's spouse requested that the patient should not have active treatment. An end of life care pathway was commenced by a consultant four hours after admission and the patient died two hours later.

The advisors questioned why was this patient was admitted to hospital and believed that they could have been cared for in the community.

Case study 19

A very elderly patient was admitted from a nursing home complaining of chest and abdominal pain following a 999 call. The patient was known to the care of the elderly department and was regularly visited by their GP. The patient had advanced dementia and ischaemic heart disease. DNAR order and an advance directive had been completed at the nursing home. The patient was promptly seen by an emergency department registrar who diagnosed generalised peritonitis due to bowel perforation. They were considered not a candidate for surgery. A consultant surgeon saw the patient shortly after admission to a surgical ward and following discussion with her relatives a DNAR proforma was completed and an end of life care pathway commenced. The patient died 24 hours later and the case was referred to the coroner. A coroner's autopsy revealed a colonic carcinoma with perforation. The patient was discussed at morbidity and mortality meeting.

The advisors were of the opinion that this patient received good hospital care with good documentation. However, in view of the existing community provision why was this patient sent to hospital as an acute admission from the nursing home?

Most patients were admitted either via the emergency department or as a referral from a GP and this proportion was the same regardless of the expectation of survival (Figure 8.2).

Case study 20

An elderly patient was admitted from home, unconscious, to the emergency department in the early hours of the morning following a 999 call by a distressed relative. The patient was receiving palliative care at home through their GP for asbestosis and mesothelioma. There was a history of increasing shortness of breath in the last 24 hours and they had been waiting for the out of hours GP service to attend

the patient's home. The patient died three hours after arrival.

Why was this patient admitted to the emergency department? The advisors considered that there was lack of community support for this patient and their family. Better arrangements should have been made for out of hours home care.

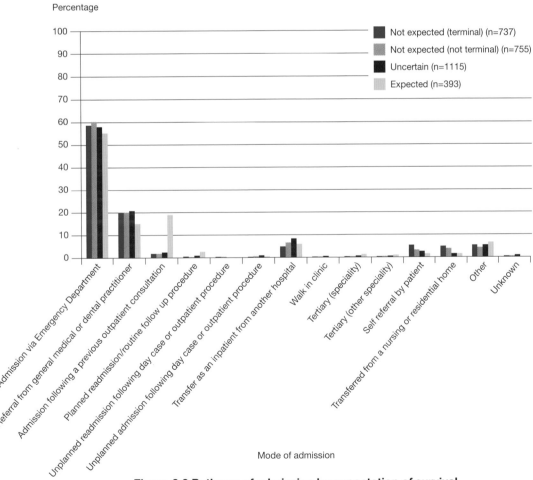

Figure 8.2 Pathway of admission by expectation of survival

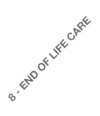

Table 8.3 Expectation to survive by medical or surgical admission

Expectation of survival	Medical		Surgical		Subtotal	Mode of admission not specified
	n	%	n	%		n
Not expected (terminal)	330	48.8	346	51.2	**676**	69
Not expected (not terminal)	432	61.9	266	38.1	**698**	62
Uncertain	527	51.4	499	48.6	**1026**	94
Expected	144	38.6	229	61.4	**373**	24
Subtotal	**1433**		**1340**		**2773**	**249**
Not answered	9		14			14
Grand Total	**1442**		**1354**			**263**

Of the medical and surgical patient admissions there were more medical patients admitted for not terminal care who were not expected to survive compared to the surgical patients of the same category (Table 8.3).

This reflects the fact that there was a greater proportion of medical patients with end stage non-cancer diseases such as chronic pulmonary disease and neurological diseases compared to inoperable surgical conditions such as a perforated diverticular disease.

In the advisors' opinion the specialty to which the patient was initially admitted was appropriate in 94% (1952/2081) of cases (insufficient data to assess in 144 cases) and this was the same proportion regardless of the expectation of survival. This indicates that the triage process which was undertaken at admission was functioning well.
It is important that patients who are expected to die and require end of life care are admitted to a ward which is suitable for their needs. In most cases this would be expected to be a general or specialist non critical care ward. However, where it could be determined, 91/739 (12.3%) of patients who were not expected to survive for not terminal care were admitted to level 3 units. This compares to 54/724 (7.5%) of patients for terminal care who were admitted to level 3 units. There may

be circumstances when patients with non survivable conditions should be cared for on an intensive care unit, for example following a rapid deterioration of an acute condition to allow the relatives to come to terms with the evolving situation. However, one has to wonder whether all these admissions to level 3 units were appropriate in view of the expected outcome of these patients.

Decision making on end of life care pathways

Early senior clinician involvement in the management of patients admitted as an emergency can improve the quality of care[61,62]. This is as much true for patients who require end of life care as it is for patients where early intervention can save life. Early decision making by a senior clinician on the limitation of treatment, the commencement of an end of life care pathway (ELCP) and the resuscitation status will expedite care.

The NCEPOD report of 2007 *"Emergency Admissions: A journey in the right direction?"*[3] identified that in approximately 16% of patients admitted as an emergency there was a delay in consultant review. In this current study the advisors considered that there was evidence of a delay in 25% (385/1553) of patients (there was insufficient data to assess in 500 cases). While the samples from the two studies are not identical they both represent admissions in a group of acutely ill patients. The original data was collected two years prior to the current sample. Consequently, it would seem that little progress has been made to ensure that patients admitted with acute conditions are reviewed by consultants at the earliest opportunity as recommended by NCEPOD and the Royal College of Physicians[5].

The advisors considered there to be a delay in assessment by a consultant in 20.9% and 23% respectively for those patients not expected to survive for terminal or not terminal care. This was somewhat better than for those patients whose survival was uncertain or they were expected to survive (Table 8.4).

Table 8.4 Delay being assessed by a consultant by expectation of survival

	Delay in consultant review					Grade not recorded/ Not answered/Unable to answer	
	Yes		No		Subtotal		Total
Expectation of survival	n	%	No	%			
Not expected (terminal)	72	20.9	272	79.1	344	137	481
Not expected (not terminal)	93	23	312	77	405	122	527
Uncertain	157	26.6	434	73.4	591	192	783
Expected	56	28.3	142	71.7	198	79	277
Subtotal	378		1160		1538	530	2068
Not answered	7		8			7	22
Grand Total	385		1168			537	2090

The advisors were asked to assess whether a clear management plan was present in the patients' case notes. In only 130/2110 (6.1%) of patients was there no evidence of a clear management plan. This is encouraging but for those patients without a clear management plan this may have affected their quality of care. In 115 cases there was insufficient data for the advisors to assess the case. Table 8.5 shows that there was little difference whether the patient was expected to survive or not and whether a management plan was in place.

In most situations where decisions regarding treatment limitation are required a discussion should take place between the health care team and the patient and or relatives. This discussion should be clearly documented in the case notes. This should occur as early as possible before clinical deterioration may render the patient unable to participate in the discussion process. If this is the case then the clinical team should have a dialogue with the patient's relatives. The GMC provides guidance on treatment limitation decision making[63]. Furthermore the responsibility of doctors to assess the mental capacity of patients in decisions on treatment options is set out in the Mental Capacity Act 2005. In the absence of an appropriate relative or close friend each hospital should have a policy for dealing with this situation[64].

In 654/2813 (23.3%) patients the clinician completing the clinical questionnaire indicated that no discussion took place on the withdrawal of treatment before the patients' death. However this question was not answered for 246/3059 (8.0%) of cases. Based on the expectation of survival of the patient Figure 8.3 shows where a discussion had taken place either with the patient or a relative. For those patients not expected to survive 16.9% (219/1293) did not have such discussions.

Table 8.5 Expectation of survival by presence of a clear management plan

	Evidence of management plan				Subtotal	Not answered	Total
	Yes		No				
Expectation of survival	n	%	No	%	n	n	n
Not expected (terminal care)	442	95.5	21	4.5	463	18	481
Not expected (not terminal)	476	93.9	31	6.1	507	20	527
Uncertain	685	93.2	50	6.8	735	48	783
Expected	242	93.1	18	6.9	260	17	277
Subtotal	1845		120		1965	103	2068
Not answered	19		1			2	22
Grand Total	1864		121			105	2090

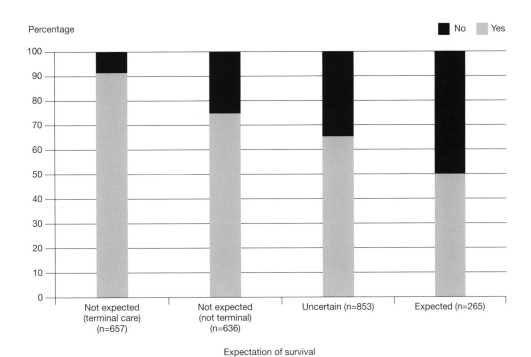

Percentage

■ No ▨ Yes

Expectation of survival

Figure 8.3 Treatment withdrawal discussed with patient and/or relative by expectation of survival on admission

For the majority of patients admitted for terminal care, discussions took place on treatment withdrawal with either the patient or relatives; in only 58/657 (8.8%) cases did this not occur. However in those patients who were for not terminal care and not expected to survive 161/636 (25.3%) there were no such discussions. It is for these patients, where death had been expected on admission, that health care teams should have had full discussions on treatment withdrawal. The fact that these did not occur is indicative of poor communication between the health care team and patients and relatives.

Use of end of life care pathways

Once the decision has been made, in discussion between the health care team, patient and or relatives, on treatment limitations the aim of the health care team should be centred on providing best end of life care. This should include:

" • *assessment of needs, planning of end of life care and regular review;*
 • *co-ordination of care;*
 • *delivery of high quality services;*
 • *care in the last days of life;*
 • *care after death.*"[59]

Various care pathways have been developed to help improve end of life care. These include the Gold Standards Framework[65], Liverpool Care Pathway[66] and Preferred Priorities for Care[67]. They also provide guidance on identifying the point at which an ELCP should commence. While these may well be an aid to patient care by providing a common framework, good quality end of life care can equally well be provided by committed and compassionate individuals who are experienced in the care of the dying. Indeed consideration should be taken to prevent the act of dying becoming overly medicalised and process driven. Perhaps the greatest value of these care pathways may be in situations were health care professionals are less confident and experienced in providing end of life care.

The use of ELCPs may be well developed by hospices, oncology units and palliative care teams, however these may be less frequently employed by health care teams in the acute hospital setting. Table 8.6 shows the number of patients who were not expected to survive who had an ELCP commenced before they died.

Table 8.6 Use of end of life care pathway for patients not expected to survive on admission.

End of life care pathway	n	%
Yes	474	33.0
No	757	52.7
Unknown	205	14.3
Subtotal	**1436**	
Not answered	69	
Grand Total	**1505**	

In only 33% (474/1436) of patients was an ELCP used. Furthermore, if these patients are grouped by whether they were for terminal or not terminal care one can see that 46.1% and 20.5% respectively had an ELCP (Table 8.7).

Table 8.7 Use of ELCP by terminal care and not terminal care patients

Expectation of survival	End of life care pathway	n	%
Not expected (terminal care)	Yes	323	46.1
	No	273	38.9
	Unknown	105	15.0
	Subtotal	**701**	
	Not answered	44	
Not expected (not terminal care)	Yes	151	20.5
	No	484	65.9
	Unknown	100	13.6
	Subtotal	**735**	
	Not answered	25	
Grand Total		**1505**	

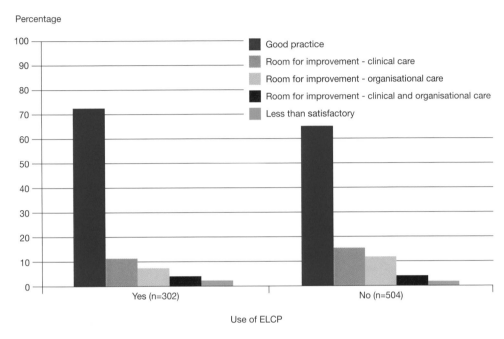

Percentage

**Figure 8.4. Overall quality of care of patients not expected to survive
who did or not have an ELCP**

As previously stated this does not necessarily indicate that every patient without an ELCP received less good care compared to those that did have an ELCP. However in those patients who did not have an ELCP, the advisors believed that overall quality of care was less good than those who had such a pathway in place (Figure 8.4). Furthermore there were examples of less than satisfactory care in patients who did not have an ELCP in use.

Not all patients that are admitted to hospital who are not expected to survive in fact die. Consequently, as previously stated, careful consideration is required on end of life decisions. However, in this study of patients that died, the fact that in a third of patients not expected to survive, an ELCP was not used would indicate that in the acute hospital setting ELCPs are not as well developed as they could be. Acute hospitals have responsibility to ensure that appropriate governance structures are in place to ensure the delivery of ELCPs.

Use of Do Not Attempt Resuscitation orders

One important component of end of life care is determination of the patient's resuscitation status. This should be fully discussed with the patient and or relatives. If it is not possible to have such a discussion the reasons should be clearly documented. The documentation of this status is frequently in the form of a DNAR order. Since 2001 all NHS Trusts are required to have a resuscitation policy which includes DNAR orders[68]. In many hospitals this is incorporated in the patients case notes as a separate a proforma which can be used to clearly indicate the current resuscitation status. The DNAR order should be reviewed regularly by the health care team as in some circumstances the resuscitation status may change.

Number of patients

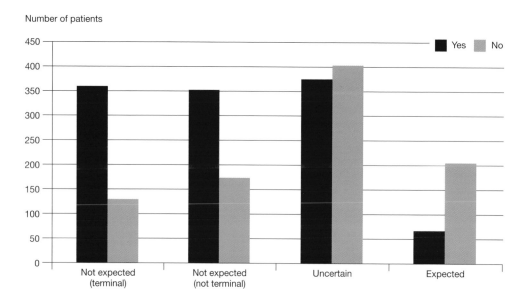

Figure 8.5 Percentage of patients who had DNAR orders by expectation of survival.

Percentage

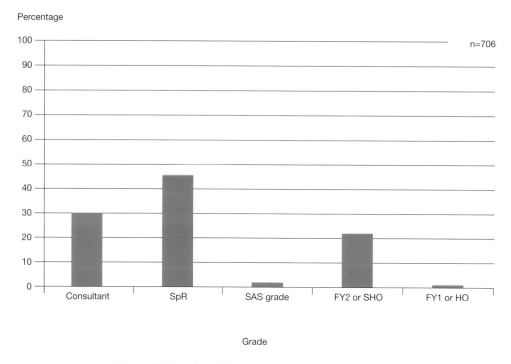

Grade

Figure 8.6 Grade of doctor who signed DNAR order

The advisors were asked to identify specific documentation within the case notes which related to end of life care. Of the 2225 patients reviewed by the advisors 1231 (55%) had a DNAR order. Of those patients not expected to survive on admission 70.4% (710/1008) had DNAR orders (Figure 8.5). The fact that 30% of patients who were expected to die on admission did not have a DNAR order is contrary to DH guidance.

Of those patients that had documentary evidence of a DNAR order in 14.6% (157/1077) no evidence could be found that the order was discussed with the patient or relative or the reason for not discussing this documented. This would be against accepted guidance from the General Medical Council[63].

The grade of the doctor who signed the DNAR order was also determined (Figure 8.6)

In the acute hospital setting, a senior member of the health care team, usually a consultant should make the final decision regarding a DNAR order[63] and decisions relating to cardiopulmonary resuscitation[69]. Their signature on the DNAR order would be indicative of this decision. However, data from this study showed that roughly a third of the DNAR orders were signed by a consultant (30.5%, 215/706), and almost half of orders (47.6%, 336/706) being signed by middle grade trainees. It is possible that a consultant was actively involved in the decision making of these DNAR orders and deputised the signing to their trainees. Or it may be that these middle grade trainees were more experienced senior registrars. However one has to question whether it is appropriate for 21.8% (154/706) of orders to be signed by SHO or FY (and HO) doctors as was found without countersigning by a consultant. In 527 cases the advisors were unable to/did not answer the grade of the clinician signing the DNAR form. One conclusion from these findings might be that the decision making regarding assessment of resuscitation status is not given adequate importance by the health care teams. If this is the case hospital trusts must ensure that health care teams receive appropriate training and guidance in this regard.

The following case study provides an example of some of the issues highlighted:

Case study 21

An elderly, independent patient was admitted via the emergency department with abdominal pain and distension. The patient was hypotensive and hypothermic. An abdominal ultrasound revealed distended loops of bowel, ascites and an enlarged liver. A CT scan showed a large carcinoma. The patient was admitted to an assessment unit under the surgeons and given intravenous fluid resuscitation. They were seen by a consultant surgeon 18 hours later and a MRI scan was considered. The patient remained hypotensive and further intravenous fluids were given. A different consultant reviewed them a day later and stated that there was a "need to discuss resuscitation status with relatives". A DNAR order was made in the notes but there was no documentary evidence of this discussion. The patient was transferred to a high dependency unit due to a persistent metabolic acidosis. The patient remained hypotensive and became progressively hypoxic. The patient then died six hours later having had hourly observations and repeated arterial blood gas analysis.

What was the clinical management intent for this patient? The advisors considered that there was poor decision making by the surgical team and any active management was likely to be futile. The most appropriate care for this patient should have been involvement of a palliative care team and commencement of an end of life care pathway. Admission to a level 2 care was inappropriate and undignified in the last hours of this patient's life.

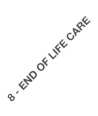

Involvement of palliative care teams

The World Health Organisation has defined palliative care as:

"an approach that improves the quality of life of patients and their families facing the problem associated with life-threatening illness, through the prevention and relief of suffering by means of early identification and impeccable assessment and treatment of pain and other problems, physical, psychosocial and spiritual"[6]

Palliative care services have developed over the last 40 years along with the hospice movement as a result of the recognition that there needs to be a compassionate and comprehensive approach to end of life care. Much of this expansion has been in the voluntary sector and there is much variation across the UK in access to palliative care services. It has been suggested that in the acute sector these services are under-represented and there is reluctance of health care professional to refer patients to palliative care teams[70].

One of the main recommendations of the DH *'End of Life Care Strategy'* is that there should be further co-ordinated development of palliative care teams both in the community and in the acute sector[59].

The advisors were asked to determine whether there was evidence of involvement of a palliative care team. Of 1478 patients reviewed in 1197(81%) there was no such involvement (this was not applicable in 541 cases and there was insufficient information to assess in 206).

These data were analysed against the clinical questionnaire and whether the patient was expected to survive or not (Table 8.8). Palliative care teams were mainly involved in patients who were for "terminal care". However, of these patients there was involvement in less than 50% of cases. Very few patients who were not expected to survive who were considered "not terminal" care, such as end stage pulmonary disease, had palliative care team involvement. While the sample of patients included in this study may not be representative of all who were admitted with palliative intent, the paucity of

Table 8.8 Involvement of palliative care team by expectation of survival.

	Palliative care involvement					
	Yes		No		Insufficient data	Total
	n	%	n	%	n	n
Not expected (terminal care)	160	43.7	206	56.3	116	482
Not expected (not terminal)	45	12.1	328	87.9	153	526
Uncertain	47	9.8	432	90.2	304	783
Expected	8	5.2	146	94.8	123	277
Subtotal	**260**		**1112**		**696**	**2068**
Not answered	2		12		8	22
Grand Total	**262**		**1124**		**704**	**2090**

input from palliative care teams may be indicative of the lack of co-ordinated end of life care in acute hospitals. In addition those patients for "not terminal care" but had end stage non cancer disease appeared to be under represented in the provision of palliative care services. Although it can be difficult to clearly identify in this group of patients the point when they are approaching the end of life, palliative care teams have as much to offer in terms of symptom control as for those with terminal cancer[59].

Inadequate involvement of palliative care teams are illustrated in the following case study:

Case study 22

A middle aged patient with advanced carcinoma and bony secondaries was admitted following a GP referral via the emergency department complaining of abdominal pain. The patient lived in a warden controlled flat and was having daily visits from a community nurse. They were diagnosed as having cholecystitis and admitted to a surgical ward. Intravenous fluids and antibiotics were commenced. The patient was not considered fit for surgery. A do not attempt resuscitation order was made in the case notes following discussion with the patient by a surgical senior house officer. The patient died two days later without further review.

The advisors were of the view that a palliative care team should have been involved. There was no end of life care pathway employed for this patient. This patient's admission could have been avoided if there had been better communication with community care. Indeed admission to a hospice would have been the best scenario for this patient.

Skills and training

There is evidence that nurses and doctors lack adequate training in end of life care. The Audit Commission found that only 18% of nurses and 29% of doctors stated that their pre-registration training covered end of life care. However in the same study health care professions were of the view that they were fairly confident in their abilities in identifying, delivering and communicating end of life care[60]. Without assessing the abilities of these professionals it is not possible to determine if their perceptions were indeed true.

The advisors reviewing the case notes in this study frequently commented that there was a lack of awareness of staff to the needs of patients nearing the end of their lives. The skills which were particularly lacking were the abilities to identify patients approaching the end of life, adequate implementation of end of life care and the ability to communicate with patients, relatives and other health care professions. An example of poor knowledge and skills of health care teams is illustrated incase study 23.

As part of the DH's 'End of Life Care Strategy' the education and training in the end of life care of medical and non-medical staff is recognised as an important area that needs to be enhanced. This should be at various levels including undergraduate, postgraduate as well as in-service and continuing professional development[61]. The National Audit Office has recommended that:

"The DH should work with the relevant professional bodies to ensure that all trainee doctors, nurses, allied health professionals, and registered social care staff receive an appropriate level of training in the delivery of end of life care"[60]

Case study 23

An elderly patient with advanced lung carcinoma was admitted under the oncologists in the early hours of the morning due to increasing shortness of breath and chest pain. The patient was seen by a medical registrar who prescribed intramuscular morphine 10 mg four hourly and a DNAR order was written in the notes. There was no documentation of any discussions with the patient or relatives. Twelve hours after admission the patient had received 30 mg of morphine and was described as drowsy by the nursing staff. The patient was reviewed by a senior house officer who prescribed intramuscular naloxone 0.4 mg as required. After administration of naloxone the patient became agitated, complained of increasing pain and died four hours later without being seen by a consultant.

The advisors considered that an end of life care pathway should have been commenced on admission. While the DNAR order was appropriate, discussions with the patient and or their relatives should have taken place and have been documented. The patient's pain control management was very poorly managed and their last hours of life would have been unimaginably distressing. There was clear lack of knowledge amongst the health care staff. This patient should have had palliative care team involvement at an early stage following admission. The advisors regarded that the lack of senior level input may have contributed to this patient's substandard end of life care pathway.

An opportunity to do this exists due to the current reviews of medical education by the GMC and the Nursing and Midwifery Council[71,72]. Furthermore the Royal Colleges need to implement recommendations on incorporating end of life care training to ensure it is a core part of training for all health care professionals and a requirement for continuing professional development[73].

Quality of end of life care management

It has been recommended that the DH needs to make an assessment of quality of care provided by end of life care services to determine the impact of the implementation of the end of life care strategy[60].

Using the NCEPOD overall quality of care tool we have subdivided the patients included in this study into their expectation of survival (Figure 8.7).

The advisors considered that 68.7% of patients not expected to survive had good practice. There was a greater proportion of good practice compared to those where survival was uncertain or expected. There were many examples of good quality care for patients at the end of their lives. However nearly a third of patients not expected to survive received less than good care. This would indicate that there is considerable room for improvement in care of patients who die in acute hospitals.

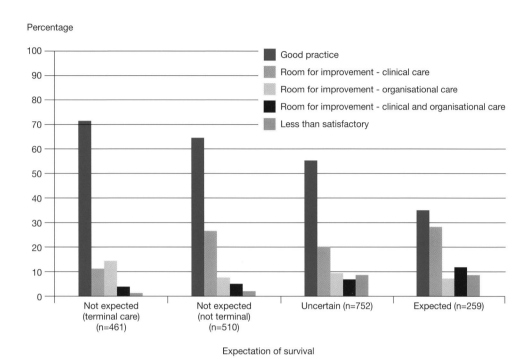

Percentage

Legend:
- Good practice
- Room for improvement - clinical care
- Room for improvement - organisational care
- Room for improvement - clinical and organisational care
- Less than satisfactory

Expectation of survival

Figure 8.7 Overall quality of care by expectation of survival

---

Case study 24

An elderly patient was admitted with increasing shortness of breath and weight loss over the previous week. There was a history of chronic pulmonary disease. The patient was anaemic with low platelets and a high white cell count. A diagnosis of acute myelomonocystic leukaemia was made. A consultant saw the patient within 12 hours of admission and discussed the poor prognosis with the patient and relatives. The patient rapidly deteriorated and a do not attempt resuscitation order was completed and an end of life care pathway was commenced. The patient died with the family in attendance.

The advisors considered that this patient received good care and were impressed with clear documentation of the discussions that the consultant had with the patient and relatives.

Case study 25

A previously independent, very elderly, patient was referred by their GP from home complaining of difficulty in swallowing. The patient was diagnosed as having suffered a stroke and following discussion with patient they wished to have "everything to be done". A nasogastric tube was passed and they were considered for a percutaneous endoscopic gastrostomy. However their condition deteriorated with loss of consciousness. A DNAR order was completed after discussion with the relatives but the patient died shortly afterwards. No end of life care ELCP was employed.

The care of this patient was considered by the advisors to be good. The patient's wishes were followed and there was good discussion with the relatives once their condition changed. Although an ELCP could have been commenced the patient received good care in the last few hours of life.

Case study 26

A middle aged patient with known metastatic carcinoma was receiving palliative care at home by their GP. Over the 24 hours prior to admission the patient became increasingly short of breath and was brought to the emergency department by a relative following discussion with the GP. A diagnosis of pneumonia was made and initially the patient wanted active treatment. They already had a DNAR order which was brought to the hospital with an advance directive. The patient was seen by a palliative care team within 24 hours of admission by which time his condition had deteriorated. Following further discussion with the patient and their relatives, active treatment was stopped and the patient was started on an end of life care pathway. The patient received good analgesia and was visited on three further occasions by palliative care team before their death 24 hours later.

The advisors considered that the patient had received good care with a high standard of documentation. There had been good communication with the GP. There was early palliative care team involvement which resulted in appropriate change in management. This case study was viewed as an excellent example of combined community and hospital end of life care.

Case study 27

A middle aged patient with chronic obstructive lung disease was admitted under the respiratory physicians. The patient continued to smoke 30 cigarettes a day. On a previous admission the patient was admitted to level 3 care and was difficult to wean from ventilatory support. On this occasion the patient was rushed to the emergency department from their home with increasing shortness of breath. They were hypoxic and hypercapneoic on maximal medical therapy. The patient was rapidly reviewed by an adult intensive care consultant and was admitted to level 2 care and commenced on non-invasive ventilatory support. Initially the patient's condition improved but 12 hours later they requested withdrawal of all active treatment. A DNAR order was completed and an end of life care ELCP commenced. The patient was seen by a palliative care team and died two hours later.

The advisors deemed that this patient had received excellent terminal care with logical endpoints which were clearly discussed and documented. There was a good ELCP which was "hard to do better than this".

A great deal of work has been done in recent years to raise the profile of end of life care and it is hoped that the DH *"End of Life Care Strategy"* will provide appropriate funding of services and support for people who are dying in the community and in hospital. Much of what is required is for those who are caring for people nearing the end of their lives to be sensitive and compassionate to the needs of the individual. This does not always necessitate complex processes of care. Indeed it would be unrealistic and inappropriate if there was a requirement that all of us need to enter an ELCP before we die.

Key findings

49.8% of patients, who died with 96 hours of admission to acute hospitals, were not expected to survive and 68.7% of these were considered to have received good practice.

The advisors considered that 5.9% of patients had an unnecessary admission to hospital and this was due to a deficiency of social and medical support in the community.

In 16.9% (219/1293) of patients who were not expected to survive on admission there was no evidence of any discussion between the health care team and either the patient or relatives on treatment limitation.

Of those patients not expected to survive on admission in only a third were end of life care pathways used and 30% did not have do not attempt resuscitation (DNAR) orders.

In 21.8% of cases DNAR orders were signed by very junior trainee doctors.

Palliative care teams were rarely involved in the care of patients who died in this study.

There were examples of where health care professionals were judged not to have the skills required to care for patients nearing the end of their lives. This was particularly so in relation to a lack of the abilities to identify patients approaching the end of life, inadequate implementation of end of life care and the poor communication with patients, relatives and other health care professions.

9 - Death certification and autopsies

Clinical questionnaire	Total population	3153
Assessment form	Total population	2302

Reporting deaths to a coroner and subsequent autopsies

It is a requirement under the Coroners Act 1988 for England and Wales[74] that deaths suspected of being violent or unnatural (e.g. potentially iatrogenic) or whose cause is unknown are reported to a coroner. This includes peri-operative and other peri-interventional deaths, although the precise criteria vary considerably across coronial jurisdictions.

From all the deaths reported to NCEPOD, we had information on 94.9% (2991/3153) of cases on what happened with respect to the coroner.

Table 9.1 Death reported to a coroner

Death reported to a coroner	n	%
Yes	1346	45.0
No	1132	37.8
Unknown	513	17.2
Subtotal	2991	
Not answered	162	
Grand Total	3153	

Table 9.2 Coroner's autopsy performed

Coroner's autopsy performed	n	%
Yes	410	30.9
No	708	53.4
Unknown	209	15.7
Subtotal	1327	
Not answered	19	
Grand Total	1346	

In this study, just under half of the deaths in hospitals were reported to a coroner (Table 9.1), which is average for all deaths in England & Wales and one third of those were investigated further with an autopsy requested by a coroner (this is less than the average overall) (Table 9.2).

Further to this, where the death was reported to the coroner, and no coronial autopsy was performed, a hospital autopsy was requested in only 19/623 cases. It was unknown or not answered whether a hospital autopsy was requested in a further 85 cases.

The clinicians completing the questionnaire indicated in 36/222 cases there were additional unexpected findings in the autopsy report. The advisors' also assessed whether the autopsies provided unexpected findings. Of the 330/1640 which could be assessed 101(36.5%) indicated that there were diseases and processes not anticipated before death (there was insufficient information to assess in 662 cases). Table 9.3 shows the more frequent categories of these unexpected autopsy findings, and some important negatives.

Table 9.3 Notable autopsy findings

Notable autopsy finding	n
Myocardial infarction/ischaemic heart disease	9
Pneumonia +/- empyema	9
Bowel ischaemia and infarction	3
Dissection of the aorta	4
Perforated gastric ulcer and peritonitis	3
Not pneumonia (as in the medical certificate of the cause of death - MCCD)	1
Not pulmonary thromboembolism (as in the MCCD)	1

Such data are entirely within the range of 'clinico-pathological discrepancies' that have been reported over the last 30 years when discussing the utility of autopsies in hospital deaths. They demonstrate information that should be fed back into the clinical audit cycle via regular mortality meetings.

Finally, the advisors were asked to comment on whether the given causes of death in MCCDs were appropriate, from the information provided on each case. In 97/929, (10%) cases where it was possible to comment, the advisor disagreed with the cause of death. Most of these differences of opinion related to the ordering of the reported 'main pathologies' versus 'comorbidities' (as in Part 2) on the MCCD. In fact, the Office for National Statistics collates data on all significant-appearing pathologies with less attention paid to the relative order than clinicians realise, as it knows that doctors are not very good at constructing logical MCCDs.

However, in 7/71 cases, the advisors considered that the case should have been reported to a coroner, and accepted for further investigation, rather than resulting in a MCCD. The reasons given included evident trauma (e.g. subdural haemorrhage), questionable bowel perforation, and unexpected death during a recovery process. With the expected passing of the Coroner and Justice Bill 2009, there will be in place a system of Medical Examiners (ME) who will scrutinise all drafted causes of death before the issuing of a MCCD, and these MEs should thus have a standardising effect on the reporting of deaths to coroners[75]. Exactly where the threshold will be set for reporting deaths in medical care will be set and, similarly, what threshold for accepting them for investigation will be followed by coroners, are yet to be determined.

1. National Confidential Enquiry into Patient Outcome and Death. 2002. Functioning as a Team. London. http://www.ncepod.org.uk/pdf/2002/02full.pdf

2. National Confidential Enquiry into Patient Outcome and Death. 2003. Who Operates When? II. London. http://www.ncepod.org.uk/pdf/2003/03full.pdf

3. National Confidential Enquiry into Patient Outcome and Death. 2007. Emergency Admissions: A journey in the right direction?. London. http://www.ncepod.org.uk/2007report1/Downloads/EA_report.pdf

4. Department of Health. 2001. Reforming Emergency Care. London. http://www.dh.gov.uk/prod_consum_dh/groups/dh_digitalassets/@dh/@en/documents/digitalasset/dh_4125520.pdf

5. The Royal College of Physicians of London. 2008. Consultant physicians working with patients. London. http://www.rcplondon.ac.uk/pubs/contents/6384bbcb-72ec-4406-b9d1-5db1724aeff2.pdf

6. World Health Organisation. Definition of palliative care. http://www.who.int/cancer/palliative/definition/en/

7. HM Government. 2009. EWTD-Surgery - e-petition response http://www.number10.gov.uk/Page20230

8. Pers. comm. Between Professor John Black, President of the Royal College of Surgeons and Alan Johnson MP.

9. The Association of Surgeons of Great Britain and Ireland. 2007. Emergency General Surgery: A consensus statement.

10. The Royal College of Surgeons of England. 2006. Centralisation and specialisation of hospital services. Bigger is not necessarily better for remote and rural communities. London.

11. The Royal College of Anaesthetists and Association of Anaesthetists of Great Britain and Ireland. 2006. Good Practice – a guide for departments of anaesthesia, critical care and pain management. Third addition. London. http://www.rcoa.ac.uk/docs/goodpractice(oct2006).pdf

12. Association of Anaesthetists of Great Britain and Ireland. 2001. Pre-operative assessment. The role of the anaesthetist. London. http://www.aagbi.org/publications/guidelines/docs/preoperativeass01.pdf

13. The Royal College of Anaesthetists. 2009. Guidelines for the provision of Anaesthetic services. London. http://www.rcoa.ac.uk/index.asp?PageID=477

14. Pager CK. Randomised controlled trial of pre-operative information to improve satisfaction with cataract surgery. Br J Ophthalmol 2005;89:10-13

15. Sills J, Wan CK. Effects of sensory and procedural information on coping with stressful medical procedures and pain: a meta analysis J Consult Clin Psychol 1989;57:372-9

16. Association of Anaesthetists of Great Britain and Ireland. 2006. Information and Consent for Anaesthesia: Revised Edition. London. http://www.aagbi.org/publications/guidelines/archive/docs/consent99.pdf

17. General Medical Council. Good Medical Practice. 2006. London. http://www.gmc-uk.org/guidance/good_medical_practice/index.asp

18. NHS Litigation Authority. 2002. Clinical Risk Management Standards. London. http://www.nhsla.com/RiskManagement/

19. Standards of Records, Kings Fund Organisation Audit.

20. Association of Anaesthetists of Great Britain and Ireland. 2007. Recommendations for standards of monitoring during anaesthesia and recovery. 4th Edition. London. http://www.aagbi.org/publications/guidelines/docs/standardsofmonitoring07.pdf

21. National Institute for Health and Clinical Excellence. 2008. Clinical Guideline 65 Inadvertent perioperative hypothermia. London. http://www.nice.org.uk/nicemedia/pdf/CG65NICEGuidance.pdf

22. Audit Commission. 2002. Acute hospital portfolio. Review of National Findings. Radiology. http://www.audit-commission.gov.uk/SiteCollectionDocuments/AuditCommissionReports/NationalStudies/Radiology_Full.pdf)

23. The Royal College of Radiologists. 2009. Standards for providing a 24 hour diagnostic radiology service. London. https://www.rcr.ac.uk/docs/radiology/pdf/BFCR(09)3_diagnostic24hr.pdf

24. National Confidential Enquiry into Patient Outcome and Death. 2007 Trauma: Who cares?. London. http://www.ncepod.org.uk/2007report2/Downloads/SIP_report.pdf

25. The Royal College of Radiologists. Standards for the communication of critical, urgent or unexpected significant radiological findings. https://www.rcr.ac.uk/docs/radiology/pdf/Stand_urgent_reports.pdf

26. European Association of Radiologists. Risk management in radiology in Europe, European Association of Radiologists. Good practice guide for European radiologists. http://www.myesr.org/html/img/pool/ESR_2006_II_GoodPractice_Web.pdf

27. National Patient Safety Agency. Safer Practice Notice 16. Early identification of failure to act on radiological imaging reports.

28. CJ Garvey, S Connolly. Radiology reporting – where does the radiologist's duty end?. Lancet 2006; 367:443-47.

29. The Royal College of Radiologists. 2007. Making the best use of Clinical Radiology services – MBUR6. http://www.rcr.ac.uk/content.aspx?PageID=995

30. National Institute for Health and Clinical Excellence. 2008. Clinical Guideline 46. Venous thromboembolism (surgical). London. www.nice.org.uk/CG466

31. National Statistics-population by age, UK. 2007. www.statistics.gov.uk/cci/nugget.asp?ID=949

32. Confidential Enquiry into Maternal and Child Health. 2006. Why Children Die-a pilot study. London. www.cemach.org.uk

33. The Royal College of Paediatrics and Child Health. 2007. Modelling the Future 1- a consultation paper on the future of children's health services. www.rcpch.ac.uk

34. National Confidential Enquiry into Patient Outcome and Death. 1999. Extremes of Age. www.ncepod.org.uk

35. New South Wales Commission for Children and Young People. 1996-2005. Trends in Child Deaths in NSW. www.kids.nsw.gov.au/documents/NSW-CDRT-10-Year-Study1.pdf

36. Lung and Asthma Information agency. The burden of respiratory disease in childhood. Fact sheet 2003/2. www.laia.ac.uk/factsheets/20012.pdf

37. Gupta R, Strachan D. The Health of Children and Young people. Chap 7. Asthma and allergic disease. www.statistics.gov.uk/children/downloads/asthma.pdf

38. Russell G. Paediatric respiratory mortality: past triumphs, future challenges. Thorax 2007 60 (12) 985-986

39. National statistics. Asthma and Allergies in children and young people. www.statistics.gov.uk/cci/nugget.asp?id=722

40. Department of Health. 2006. "Pneumococcal vaccine added to the childhood immunisation programme. www.dh.gov.uk

41. Kyaw et al. Effect of introduction of Pneumococcal conjugated vaccine on drug resistant Strep pneuomiae infection. NEJM 2006; 44: 1455-1463

42. Immunisation against infectious diseases-The Green Book. 3rd edition 2006. Gateway 7523. www.dh.gov.uk

43. The Royal College of Paediatrics and Child Health. 2008. Supporting Reconfiguration-a framework for standards. www.rcpch.ac.uk

44. The Royal College of Paediatrics and Child Health. 2007. Modelling the Future 2-Reconfiguration and workforce estimates. www.rcpch.ac.uk

45. Services for Children in Emergency Departments-Intercollegiate committee for services for children in emergency departments. April 2007. www.rcpch.ac.uk

46. National report: Paediatric intensive care audit network Jan 2005-Dec 2007. Pub June 2008. University of Leeds and Leicester. ISBN 978 0 8531 62759. www.picanet.ac.uk

47. Epidemiology of critically ill children in England and Wales: incidence, mortality, deprivation and ethnicity. Arch Dis Child 2009;94: 210-215.

48. Department of Health. 2006. The acutely or critically sick or injured child in the DGH: A team response. Gateway 6369. www.dh.gov.uk/publications

49. National Institute for Health and Clinical Excellence. 2007. Clinical Guideline 47. Feverish illness in children. www.guidance.nice.org.uk/CG47

50. Duncan H, Hutchison J, Parshuram CS. The Paediatric Early Warning system score, a severity of illness score to predict urgent medical need in hospitalized children. J Crit Care 2006; 21(3): 271-8.

51. Formulae for weight estimation in resuscitation: is the current formula still valid ? Luscombe M, Owens B. Archives of Disease of Childhood, 2007;92: 412-5

52. So Ty et al. Evaluation of accuracy of different methods used to estimate weight in the paediatric population. Pediatrics, June 2009 e 1045-51.

53. Department of Health. 2007. Palliative Care Services for Children and young People in England-an independent review for the Secretary of State for Health. www.dh.gov.uk/publications

54. HM Government. 2006. Working Together to Safeguard Children: a guide to interagency working to safeguard and promote the health of children. www.everychildmatters.gov.uk

55. HM Government. 2006. Working Together to Safeguard Children: a guide to interagency working to safeguard and promote the health of children. www.everychildmatters.gov.uk

56. Gomes B, Higginson IJ. Where people die (1974–2030): Past trends, future projections and implications for care. Palliative Medicine 2008; 22: 33–41.

57. Griffiths C, Brock A. Twentieth century mortality trends in England and Wales. Health Stat Quarterly 2003; 18:5-17.

58. National End of Life Care Programme. http://www.endoflifecareforadults.nhs.uk/eolc/

59. Department of Health. 2008. End of Life Care Strategy. London. http://www.dh.gov.uk/en/Publicationsandstatistics/Publications/PublicationsPolicyAndGuidance/DH_086277

60. National Audit Office. 2008. End of Life Care. Stationery Office London. http://www.nao.org.uk/publications/0708/end_of_life_care.aspx

61. National Patient Safety Agency. 2007. Safer care for the acutely ill patient: learning from critical incidents.

62. National Institute for Health and Clinical Excellence. 2007. Clinical Guideline 50. Acutely ill patients in hospital. Recognition of and response to illness in adults in hospital. London. http://guidance.nice.org.uk/CG50/NiceGuidance/pdf/English

63. General Medical Council. 2002. Withholding and withdrawing life-prolonging treatments: Good practice in decision making. 2002 http://www.gmc-uk.org/guidance/current/library/witholding_lifeprolonging_guidance.asp,

64. Department of Health. 2007. Independent Mental Capacity Advocate service. http://www.dh.gov.uk/en/SocialCare/Deliveringadultsocialcare/MentalCapacity/IMCA/index.htm

65. The Gold Standards Framework. http://www.goldstandardsframework.nhs.uk/GSFOtherSettings/AcuteHospitalSettings/

66. The Marie Curie Palliative Care Institute. Liverpool Care Pathway for the Dying Patient. http://www.mcpcil.org.uk/liverpool-care-pathway/index.htm

67. National End of Life Care Programme. Preferred priorities for care. http://www.endoflifecareforadults.nhs.uk/eolc/ppc.htm

68. Department of Health. 2000. Resuscitation policy (HSC 2000/028). London. http://www.dh.gov.uk/en/Publicationsandstatistics/Lettersandcirculars/Healthservicecirculars/DH_4004244

69. A joint statement from the British Medical Association, the Resuscitation Council (UK) and the Royal College of Nursing. 2007. Decisions relating to cardiopulmonary resuscitation. http://www.resus.org.uk/pages/dnar.pdf

70. Sheffield Palliative Care Studies Group. Improving Access to Palliative Care. http://www.access2pallcare.org.uk/index.shtml

71. General Medical Council. 2009. Tomorrow's Doctors: A draft for consultation. http://www.gmc-uk.org/education/undergraduate/news_and_projects/Tomorrow_s_Doctors_2009_-_a_draft_for_consultation.pdf

72. Nursing and Midwifery Council. Review of pre-registration nursing education. http://www.nmc-uk.org/aArticle.aspx?ArticleID=3566

73. Palliative care services: meeting the needs of patients Report of a Working Party RCP London 2007. http://www.rcplondon.ac.uk/pubs/contents/ec579e02-64fd-4f36-bb5d-5159a276077f.pdf).

74. Coroners Act 1988. http://www.opsi.gov.uk/acts/acts1988/ukpga_19880013_en_1

75. Coroner and Justice Bill. http://services.parliament.uk/bills/2008-09/coronersandjustice.html

Appendices

Appendix 1

Glossary

AICU	Adult Intensive Care Unit
ASA	American Society of Anesthesiologists
CCST	Certificate of Completion of Specialist Training
CCT	Certificate of Completion of Training
CT	Computed Tomography (scan)
DH	Department of Health
DNAR	Do Not Attempt Resuscitation
DVT	Deep Vein Thrombosis
ECG	Electrocardiogram
ED	Emergency Department
ELCP	End of Life Care Pathway
EWTD	European Working Time Directive
FY	Foundation Year
GCS	Glasgow Coma Score
GMC	General Medical Council
GP	General Practitioner
HO	House Officer
LMWH	Low Molecular Weight Heparin
MCCD	Medical Certificate of Cause of Death
ME	Medical Examiner
NICE	National Institute for Health and Clinical Excellence
OPCS	Office of Population Censuses and Surveys
PCT	Primary Care Trust
PICU	Paediatric Intensive Care Unit
PRHO	Pre Registration House Officer
SHO	Senior House Officer
SpR	Specialist Registrar
SAS	Staff Grade and Associate Specialist
VTE	Venous Thromboembolism

Appendix 2

Advisors and acknowledgements

Alison Rawle	Nurse Consultant	Emergency Medicine
Andrew Fordyce	Consultant	Oral and Maxillofacial Surgeon
Andrew Knowles	Consultant	Anaesthetist
Anthony Jones	Consultant	Cardiologist
Carl Stevenson	Consultant	Oral and Maxillofacial Surgeon
Carl Waldmann	Consultant	Anaesthesia and Critical Care
Charles van Heyningen	Consultant	Chemical Pathologist and Clinical Director for Pathology
Charlotte Daman Willems	Consultant	Paediatrician
Chris Chandler	Consultant	Gynaecologist
Chris Maimaris	Consultant	Emergency Medicine
Christopher Scott	Consultant	Anaesthesia and Critical Care
Daren P Forward	Consultant	Trauma & Orthopaedic Surgeon
David Feuer	Consultant	Palliative Medicine
David Goldhill	Consultant	Anaesthesia and Critical Care
David Hughes	Consultant	Peri-op & Critical Care Services
David John	Consultant	ENT Surgeon
Deepak Gupta	Consultant	ENT Surgeon
Deirdre Connors	Clinical Matron	Medicine and Elderly Care
Duncan Watson	Consultant	Critical Care Medicine
Edward Seward	Consultant	Gastroenterologist, Endoscopy Unit
Elaine Lennan	Consultant Nurse	Oncology
Elizabeth Haxby	Lead Clinician - Clinical Risk	Anaesthetist
Emma Greig	Consultant	Physician and Gastroenterologist
Eurem Matthews	Consultant	Paediatrician
Frances Calman	Consultant	Clinical Oncologist
Gareth John	Consultant	ENT Surgeon
Geir Grotte	Honorary Consultant	Cardiothoracic Surgeon
George Noble	Consultant	Physician
Graham Briars	Consultant	Paediatrician
Gwyn Seymour	Consultant	Old Age Medicine
Harry Ward	Consultant	Paediatric Surgeon
Helen Cattermole	Consultant	Trauma & Orthopaedic Surgeon
Hugh Markus	Professor	Neurology
Ian Barrison	Consultant	Physician/Gastroenterologist
Ian Botterill	Consultant	Colorectal Surgeon

Jane Wainwright	Consultant	Neurology
Jayaraman Thiagarajan	Consultant	Anaesthesia and Critical Care
Jeremy Sharp	Consultant	ENT Surgeon
Joerg Kuehne	Consultant	Anaesthetist
John Phillips	Specialist Registrar	Otolaryngology, Head & Neck Surgery
Jonathan Argall	Consultant	Emergency Medicine
Jonathan Frappell	Consultant	Obstetrics and Gynaecology
Jonathan Nicoll	Consultant	Clinical Oncologist
Kath Thorley	Clinical Standards Manager	Clinical Governance
Krish Ravi	Consultant	Upper GI and Laparoscopic surgeon
Laurence Newman	Consultant	Oral and Maxillofacial Surgeon
Linda Walker	Senior Nurse	Operating Theatres
Mahir Hamad	Consultant	Acute Physician
Mansur Reza	Consultant	Physician in Acute and General [Integrated] Medicine
Mario Calleja	Consultant	Anaesthetist
Mark Sacks	Consultant	Anaesthetist
Mary-Anne Morris	Consultant	Paediatrician
Matthew Clarke	Charge Nurse/Team Leader	Emergency Theatres
Matthew Wise	Consultant	Critical Care Medicine
Maurice Cohen	Consultant	Clinical director for elderly medicine
Michael Crawford	Consultant	Medical Oncologist
Michael S. Norell	Consultant	Cardiologist
Mohan Thomas	Consultant	Acute Physician
Morgan McMonagle	Specialist Registrar	General and Vascular Surgery
Morganaden Moorghen	Consultant	Histopathologist
Nandu Thalange	Consultant	Paediatrician
Natasha Robinson	Consultant	Anaesthetist
Neil Kitchen	Consultant	Neurosurgery & Head of Victor Horsley Department of Neurosurgery
Neil Rothwell	Consultant	Urological Surgeon
Nicholas Barron	Consultant	Anaesthetist
Nicholas Crombie	Consultant	Anaesthetist
Nick Everitt	Consultant	General and Upper Gastrointestinal Surgery
Norman Johnson	Consultant	Respiratory Physician

Norman McWhinney	Consultant	Obstetrics and Gynaecology
Pam Beacher	Clinical Audit Manager	Clinical Audit
Patrick Dill-Russell	Consultant	Anaesthetist
Paul Farquhar-Smith	Consultant	Anaesthesia and Critical Care
Pervaiz Iqbal	Consultant	Consultant Physician/Hypertension Specialist
Peter McQuillan	Consultant	Anaesthesia and Critical Care
Pyda Venkatesh	Consultant	Anaesthesia and Critical Care
Richard Elliott	Consultant	Anaesthetist
Richard J Harding	Consultant	Anaesthesia and Critical Care
Robert Banks	Consultant	Oral and Maxillofacial Surgeon
Robert Robinson	Consultant	GIM, Diabetes and Endocrinology
Roger Slater	Consultant	Anaesthesia and Critical Care
Ruth Spencer	Consultant	Anaesthetist
Sanjay Shah	Consultant	Palliative Medicine
Sath Nag	Consultant	Acute Physician
Sean Preston	Consultant	Gastroenterologist and General Physician
Shanti Soysa	Consultant	Emergency Medicine
Sharon Greasley	Project Manager/Theatre Manager	Theatre
Sharon Mooney	Consultant Nurse	Critical Care Medicine
Simon Chapman	Consultant	Emergency Medicine
Stephen D'Souza	Consultant	Interventional radiologist
T Prakash Rudra	Consultant	Geriatric Medicine
Terry Jones	Consultant	Histopathologist
Tina Sajjanhar	Consultant	Paediatrician
Virginia Sams	Consultant	Histopathologist
William Bernal	Consultant	Liver Intensive Care Medicine

Appendix 3

Trust participation

NCEPOD would like to thank the following Trusts for their participation:

Abertawe Bro Morgannwg University NHS Trust
Aintree Hospitals NHS Foundation Trust
Airedale NHS Trust
Alder Hey Children's NHS Foundation Trust
Ashford & St Peter's Hospital NHS Trust
Aspen Healthcare
Barking, Havering & Redbridge University Hospitals NHS Trust
Barnet and Chase Farm Hospitals NHS Trust
Barnsley Hospital NHS Foundation Trust
Barts and The London NHS Trust
Basildon & Thurrock University Hospitals NHS Foundation Trust
Basingstoke & North Hampshire Hospitals NHS Foundation Trust
Bedford Hospital NHS Trust
Benenden Hospital
Belfast Health and Social Care Trust
Birkdale Clinic
Birmingham Children's Hospital NHS Foundation Trust
Birmingham Women's Healthcare NHS Trust
Blackpool, Fylde and Wyre Hospitals NHS Foundation Trust
BMI Healthcare
Bolton Hospitals NHS Trust
Bradford Teaching Hospitals NHS Foundation Trust
Brighton and Sussex University Hospitals NHS Trust
Bromley Hospitals NHS Trust
Buckinghamshire Hospitals NHS Trust
BUPA Cromwell Hospital
Burton Hospitals NHS Foundation Trust
Calderdale & Huddersfield NHS Foundation Trust

Cambridge University Hospitals NHS Foundation Trust
Cardiff & Vale NHS Trust
Care UK
Central Manchester University Hospitals NHS Foundation Trust
Chelsea & Westminster Healthcare NHS Trust
Chesterfield Royal Hospital NHS Foundation Trust
City Hospitals Sunderland NHS Foundation Trust
Clatterbridge Centre for Oncology NHS Trust
Colchester Hospital University NHS Foundation Trust
Countess of Chester Hospital NHS Foundation Trust
County Durham and Darlington NHS Foundation Trust
County Durham Primary Care Trust
Covenant Healthcare Limited
Cwm Taf NHS Trust
Dartford & Gravesham NHS Trust
Derby Hospitals NHS Foundation Trust
Doncaster and Bassetlaw Hospitals NHS Foundation Trust
Dorset County Hospital NHS Foundation Trust
Dudley Group of Hospitals NHS Trust
Ealing Hospital NHS Trust
East & North Hertfordshire NHS Trust
East Cheshire NHS Trust
East Kent Hospitals University NHS Foundation Trust
East Kent Medical Services
East Lancashire Hospitals NHS Trust
East Sussex Hospitals NHS Trust
Epsom and St Helier University Hospitals NHS Trust
Fairfield Independent Hospital
Frimley Park Hospitals NHS Trust
Gateshead Health NHS Foundation Trust
George Eliot Hospital NHS Trust
Gloucestershire Hospitals NHS Foundation Trust
Great Ormond Street Hospital for Children NHS Trust

Great Western Hospitals NHS Foundation Trust

Guy's & St Thomas' NHS Foundation Trust

Gwent Healthcare NHS Trust

Harrogate and District NHS Foundation Trust

HCA International

Health & Social Services, States of Guernsey

Heart of England NHS Foundation Trust

Heatherwood & Wexham Park Hospitals NHS
Foundation Trust

Hereford Hospitals NHS Trust

Hillingdon Hospital NHS Trust

Hinchingbrooke Health Care NHS Trust

Homerton University Hospital NHS Foundation Trust

Hospital of St John and St Elizabeth

Hull & East Yorkshire Hospitals NHS Trust

Hywel Dda NHS Trust

Imperial College Healthcare NHS Trust

Ipswich Hospital NHS Trust

Isle of Man Department of Health & Social Security

Isle of Wight NHS Primary Care Trust

James Paget Healthcare NHS Trust

Kettering General Hospital NHS Trust

King Edward VII's Hospital Sister Agnes

King's College Hospital NHS Foundation Trust

Kingston Hospital NHS Trust

Lancashire Teaching Hospitals NHS Foundation Trust

Leeds Teaching Hospitals NHS Trust (The)

Lewisham Hospital NHS Trust

Liverpool Heart and Chest Hospital NHS Trust

Liverpool Women's Hospital NHS Trust

London Clinic

Luton and Dunstable Hospital NHS Foundation Trust

Maidstone and Tunbridge Wells NHS Trust

Mayday Health Care NHS Trust

Medway NHS Trust

Mid Cheshire Hospitals NHS Trust

Mid Staffordshire NHS Foundation Trust

Mid Yorkshire Hospitals NHS Trust

Mid Essex Hospital Services NHS Trust

Milton Keynes Hospital NHS Foundation Trust

Netcare Healthcare UK Ltd

New Victoria Hospital

Newcastle upon Tyne Hospitals NHS Foundation Trust

Newham University Hospital NHS Trust

Norfolk & Norwich University Hospital NHS Trust

North Bristol NHS Trust

North Cumbria Acute Hospitals NHS Trust

North Middlesex University Hospital NHS Trust

North Tees and Hartlepool NHS Foundation Trust

North Wales NHS Trust

North West London Hospitals NHS Trust

North West Wales NHS Trust

Northampton General Hospital NHS Trust

Northern Devon Healthcare NHS Trust

Northern Health & Social Care Trust

Northern Lincolnshire & Goole Hospitals Trust

Northumbria Healthcare NHS Foundation Trust

Nottingham University Hospitals NHS Trust

Nuffield Health

Nuffield Orthopaedic Centre NHS Trust

Oxford Radcliffe Hospital NHS Trust

Papworth Hospital NHS Foundation Trust

Pennine Acute Hospitals NHS Trust (The)

Peterborough & Stamford Hospitals NHS
Foundation Trust

Plymouth Hospitals NHS Trust

Poole Hospital NHS Trust

Portsmouth Hospitals NHS Trust

Princess Alexandra Hospital NHS Trust

Princess Mary's Hospital

Queen Elizabeth Hospital NHS Trust

Queen Mary's Sidcup NHS Trust

Queen Victoria Hospital NHS Foundation Trust

Ramsay Health Care UK

Robert Jones and Agnes Hunt Orthopaedic
& District Hospital

Royal Berkshire NHS Foundation Trust

Royal Bournemouth and Christchurch Hospitals
NHS Trust

Royal Brompton and Harefield NHS Trust

Royal Cornwall Hospitals NHS Trust

Royal Devon and Exeter NHS Foundation Trust

Royal Free Hampstead NHS Trust
Royal Liverpool & Broadgreen University Hospitals NHS Trust
Royal Marsden NHS Foundation Trust (The)
Royal National Hospital for Rheumatic Diseases NHS Trust
Royal National Orthopaedic Hospital NHS Trust
Royal Orthopaedic Hospital NHS Foundation Trust
Royal Surrey County Hospital NHS Trust
Royal United Hospital Bath NHS Trust
Royal Wolverhampton Hospitals NHS Trust (The)
Salford Royal Hospitals NHS Foundation Trust
Salisbury Foundation NHS Trust
Sandwell and West Birmingham Hospitals NHS Trust
Scarborough and North East Yorkshire Health Care NHS Trust
Sheffield Children's NHS Foundation Trust
Sheffield Teaching Hospitals NHS Foundation Trust
Sherwood Forest Hospitals NHS Trust
Shrewsbury and Telford Hospitals NHS Trust
South Devon Healthcare NHS Foundation Trust
South Downs Health NHS Trust
South Eastern Health & Social Care Trust
South Tees Hospitals NHS Trust
South Tyneside NHS Foundation Trust
South Warwickshire General Hospitals NHS Trust
Southampton University Hospitals NHS Trust
Southend University Hospital NHS Foundation Trust
Southern Health & Social Care Trust
Southport and Ormskirk Hospitals NHS Trust
Spire Healthcare
St Anthony's Hospital
St George's Healthcare NHS Trust
St Helens and Knowsley Teaching Hospitals NHS Trust
St Joseph's Hospital
States of Jersey Health & Social Services
Stockport NHS Foundation Trust
Surrey & Sussex Healthcare NHS Trust
Tameside Hospital NHS Foundation Trust
Taunton & Somerset NHS Foundation Trust
The Christie NHS Foundation Trust

The Horder Centre
The Hospital Management Trust
The London Oncology Clinic
The Queen Elizabeth Hospital King's Lynn NHS Trust
The Rotherham NHS Foundation Trust
The Walton Centre NHS Foundation Trust
Ulster Independent Clinic
Trafford Healthcare NHS Trust
United Lincolnshire Hospitals NHS Trust
University Hospital of South Manchester NHS Foundation Trust
University College London Hospitals NHS Foundation Trust
University Hospital Birmingham NHS Foundation Trust
University Hospital of North Staffordshire NHS Trust
University Hospitals Coventry and Warwickshire NHS Trust
University Hospitals of Bristol NHS Foundation Trust
University Hospitals of Leicester NHS Trust
University Hospitals of Morecambe Bay NHS Trust
Velindre NHS Trust
Walsall Hospitals NHS Trust
Warrington & Halton Hospitals NHS Foundation Trust
West Hertfordshire Hospitals NHS Trust
West Middlesex University Hospital NHS Trust
West Suffolk Hospitals NHS Trust
Western Health & Social Care Trust
Western Sussex Hospitals NHS Trust
Weston Area Health Trust
Whipps Cross University Hospital NHS Trust
Whittington Hospital NHS Trust
Winchester & Eastleigh Healthcare NHS Trust
Wirral University Teaching Hospital NHS Foundation Trust
Worcestershire Acute Hospitals
Wrightington, Wigan & Leigh NHS Foundation Trust
Yeovil District Hospital NHS Foundation Trust
York Hospitals NHS Foundation Trust

Appendix 4

Corporate structure

The National Confidential Enquiry into Patient Outcome and Death (NCEPOD) is an independent body to which a corporate commitment has been made by the Medical and Surgical Colleges, Associations and Faculties related to its area of activity. Each of these bodies nominates members on to NCEPOD's Steering Group.

Steering Group as at 5th November 2009

Dr D Whitaker	Association of Anaesthetists of Great Britain and Ireland
Mr T Bates	Association of Surgeons of Great Britain & Ireland
Mr J Wardrope	College of Emergency Medicine
Dr S Bridgman	Faculty of Public Health Medicine
Professor Ravi Mahajan	Royal College of Anaesthetists
Dr P Nightingale	Royal College of Anaesthetists
Dr B Ellis	Royal College of General Practitioners
Ms M McElligott	Royal College of Nursing
Dr T Falconer	Royal College of Obstetricians and Gynaecologists
Mrs M Wishart	Royal College of Ophthalmologists
Dr I Doughty	Royal College of Paediatrics and Child Health
Dr R Dowdle	Royal College of Physicians
Professor T Hendra	Royal College of Physicians
Dr M Armitage	Royal College of Physicians
Dr M Clements	Royal College of Physicians
Dr S McPherson	Royal College of Radiologists
Mr B Rees	Royal College of Surgeons of England
Mr M Parker	Royal College of Surgeons of England
Mr D Mitchell	Faculty of Dental Surgery, Royal College of Surgeons of England
Dr M Osborn	Royal College of Pathologists
Ms S Panizzo	Patient Representative
Mrs M Wang	Patient Representative

Observers

Mrs C Miles	Institute of Healthcare Management
Dr R Palmer	Coroners' Society of England and Wales
Mrs H Burton	Scottish Audit of Surgical Mortality
Dr K Cleary	National Patient Safety Agency
Ms R Brown	National Patient Safety Agency
Professor P Littlejohns	National Institute for Health and Clinical Excellence

NCEPOD is a company, limited by guarantee
(Company number: 3019382) and a registered charity
(Charity number: 1075588), managed by Trustees.

Trustees

Chairman	Professor T Treasure
Treasurer	Professor G T Layer
	Professor M Britton
	Professor J H Shepherd
	Mr M A M S Leigh
	Dr D Justins
Company Secretary	Dr M Mason

Clinical Co-ordinators

The Steering Group appoint a Lead Clinical Co-ordinator
for a defined tenure. In addition there are seven Clinical
Co-ordinators who work on each study. All Co-ordinators
are engaged in active academic/clinical practice (in the
NHS) during their term of office.

Lead Clinical Co-ordinator	Dr G Findlay (Intensive Care)
Clinical Co-ordinators	Dr D G Mason (Anaesthesia)
	Dr K Wilkinson (Anaesthesia)
	Dr A Goodwin (Anaesthesia)
	Dr J Stewart (Medicine)
	Professor S B Lucas (Pathology)
	Mr I C Martin (Surgery)
	Professor MJ Gough (Surgery)

Appendix 5

Supporting organisations

The organisations that provided funding to cover the cost of this study:

National Patient Safety Agency
Department of Health, Social Services and Public Safety
(Northern Ireland)
Aspen Healthcare
BMI Healthcare
Classic Hospitals
Covenant Healthcare Ltd
East Kent Medical Services Ltd
Fairfield Independent Hospital
HCA International
Hospital of St John and St Elizabeth
Isle of Man Health and Social Security Department
King Edward VII's Hospital Sister Agnes
Netcare Healthcare UK Ltd
New Victoria Hospital
Nuffield Health
Ramsay Health Care UK
Spire Health Care
St Anthony's Hospital
St Joseph's Hospital
States of Guernsey Board of Health
States of Jersey, Health and Social Services
The Benenden Hospital Trust
The Horder Centre
The Hospital Management Trust
The London Clinic
The London Oncology Clinic
Ulster Independent Clinic

The professional organisations that support our work and who constitute our Steering Group:

Association of Anaesthetists of Great Britain and Ireland
Association of Surgeons of Great Britain and Ireland
College of Emergency Medicine
Coroners' Society of England and Wales
Faculty of Dental Surgery of the Royal College of Surgeons of England
Faculty of Public Health of the Royal College of Physicians of the UK
Institute of Healthcare Management
Royal College of Anaesthetists
Royal College of Child Health and Paediatrics
Royal College of General Practitioners
Royal College of Nursing
Royal College of Obstetricians and Gynaecologists
Royal College of Ophthalmologists
Royal College of Pathologists
Royal College of Physicians of London
Royal College of Radiologists
Royal College of Surgeons of England

DISCLAIMER
This work was undertaken by NCEPOD, which received funding for this report from the National Patient Safety Agency. The views expressed in this publication are those of the authors and not necessarily those of the Agency.